The Ultimate Metabolic Plan©

Uncovering and Conquering the Roadblocks to Weight Loss

By Dr Cobi Slater, PhD, DNM, RHT, RNCP, ROHP

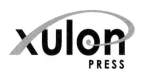

Copyright © 2015 by Dr Cobi Slater, PhD, DNM, RHT, RNCP, ROHP

The Ultimate Metabolic Plan©
Uncovering and Conquering the Roadblocks to Weight Loss
by Dr Cobi Slater, PhD, DNM, RHT, RNCP, ROHP

Printed in the United States of America

ISBN 9781498423243

All rights reserved solely by the author. The author guarantees all contents are original and do not infringe upon the legal rights of any other person or work. No part of this book may be reproduced in any form without the permission of the author. The views expressed in this book are not necessarily those of the publisher.

This book is not intended as a substitute for the medical advice of physicians. The reader should regularly consult a physician in matters relating to his/her health and particularly with respect to any symptoms that may require diagnosis or medical attention.

www.xulonpress.com

Dedication and Acknowledgements

This book is dedicated to the many people who are frustrated with the roadblocks that get in the way of their weight loss. Many of you have been seeking optimal health and weight loss but have been faced with continual disappointment due to hidden underlying causes that have been overlooked for years. May the pages of this book help to bless you with long lasting health and wellness.

Thank you to my Mom who selflessly continues to assist me in achieving my goals. Your name belongs on the cover of every book I have written as my editor and co-author. Thank you for sitting beside me for countless hours helping the words come to life on each and every page. To my Dad, you are truly an amazing man who blesses me in countless ways. Finally, to the loves of my life, Garry, Dane and Kade-I thank God for each of you and for this Slater family journey that we are on together.

Table of Contents

Metabolic Roadblocks	9
Liver Toxicity and Weight Gain	11
Stress and the Adrenals	29
The Thyroid Connection and Weight Gain	57
Estrogen Dominance	71
Food Allergies	88
The Hidden Yeast Issue - Candida	102
The Sleep Connection	126
The Detrimental Effects of Sugar	135
Insulin Resistance	142
Medications that Cause Weight Gain	152
Top Lab Tests to Uncover Hidden Road Blocks to Weight Loss and Optimal Health	157
Supplements for Metabolic Health	170
The Metabolic Plan	173
• Organic Foods	174
• The Good, the Bad and the Ugly- Fats	175
• Replacing Foods	176
• Tips for Dining out	177

- Hydration 179
- The Ultimate Metabolic Plan 181

The Maui Cleanse 184

The Metabolic Menu Plan 190

Foods to Avoid 194

Foods to Consume 196

The Metabolic Meal Plans 199

Recipes for Metabolic Health 205

The Metabolic Plan Recipes 215

Appendix 283
- Recommended Supplements 283
- Recommended Lab Testing 289
- Helpful Nutrition Websites 290

Bibliography 291

Metabolic Roadblocks

Obesity is one of the most tragic, costly and preventable public health problems. The epidemic of obesity drains the economy and costs billions of dollars annually in direct medical expenses, disability and lost productivity and together with a sedentary lifestyle, contributes to over three hundred thousand deaths each year. Next to smoking, obesity is the second leading cause of preventable death in the United States. According to the results of The National Health and Nutrition Examination Survey 111, one in three North American adults is obese. The number of obese children doubled from 1960 to 1991. Obesity in North America has long been considered an issue of cosmetics and poor self-control, much lower on the scale of importance in comparison to the needs of developing countries. This negligence allowed obesity to run rampant in North American society, gorging on our affluence and economic prosperity.[1]

For many people losing weight is much more than just cutting calories and exercising more. The age old theory of weight loss being no more than calories in versus calories out has been disproved by the masses. Many people eat incredibly clean and are enslaved to exercise 6 days a week and despite this are continually frustrated by the lack movement on the scale. Discouragement and disappointment easily sets in and the white towel is thrown in until the next fad diet comes alone and the cycle continues. Weight loss resistance is becoming more and more prevalent as the underlying reasons for sluggish metabolisms are overlooked.

---

[1] The Ultimate Hormone Balancing Guidebook- Dr Cobi Slater, PhD, DNM, RHT, RNCP

We all have a unique set of genetics and internal circumstances that will dictate our body's ability or inability to achieve a healthy weight. Weight loss resistance occurs when the body's internal balancing system is thrown off by a variety of hidden roadblocks that hinder the body from purging its protective layer. These roadblocks can include a poorly functioning liver, chronic stress, food allergies, estrogen dominance, adrenal fatigue, low thyroid function, insulin resistance, poor sleep and certain medications, all of which can prevent a person from achieving weight loss.

Discovering and conquering which roadblocks are the underlying root cause of weight loss resistance is the key to living a completely balanced and healthy lifestyle without weight fluctuations.

Liver Toxicity and Weight Gain

A seldom discussed yet extremely important aspect of weight loss is liver function. The liver is the chief operator of detoxification in the body. In our modern day society, many of our foods are laden with hidden toxins and void of nutrients. Many fad diets cause the liver to work overtime in an attempt to keep up with the high fat and nutritionally void foods and weight loss gimmicks. This eventually causes the person to gain more weight in the end as the demand on the liver is too high. Throughout this process, the liver literally becomes more and more sluggish in function and eventually becomes "fatty". Once a liver has reached the fatty stage, the function is extremely impaired and weight loss becomes an impossibility. The liver's job of detoxifying blood and metabolizing fat is compromised and the metabolism greatly slows.

The liver is a complex and unique organ, serving many functions crucial to sustaining life. From circulation to digestion, it is constantly processing blood for use by the rest of the body.

The liver is the largest internal organ in the human body, weighing three to four pounds. The rich supply of blood flowing through it causes its dark red color and glossy appearance. Sometimes called "The Great Chemical Factory," the liver neutralizes harmful toxins and wastes, stores glycogen (a blood-sugar regulator), amino acids, protein and fat.

Environmental toxins and over-processed foods which are infused with many unnatural chemicals leave the liver at great risk for contamination. If the liver is not functioning well, a hazardous buildup of toxins may occur.

From its sheltered position in the abdominal cavity, the liver filters blood and performs many functions vital to health including:

1. **Circulation:** The liver stores and regulates the blood in the body and is responsible for nourishing every cell. The liver transfers blood from the portal vein to the systemic circulation.
2. **Excretion:** The liver is responsible for the formation and secretion of bile for digestion and cleansing of blood. It removes ammonia from the blood and excretes substances filtered from the blood such as heavy metals or dyes.
3. **Metabolism:** Manufacture and storage of many nutrients such as glucose and vitamins occurs in the liver. The metabolism of carbohydrates, proteins, lipids (fat), minerals and vitamins is also a part of the liver's contribution to metabolism.
4. **Protection and detoxification:** The removal of foreign bodies from the blood (phagocytosis) and detoxification by conjugation, methylation, oxidation and reduction are some of the liver's main functions.
5. **Production:** The formation of urea, serum albumin, glycogen, and blood coagulating proteins such as prothrombin, fibrinogen and heparin occurs in the liver. The destruction of erythrocyte (red blood cells) also occurs in the liver. The liver regulates blood sugar levels and stores the balanced amount of sugar as glycogen for future energy usage.
6. **Regulation of hormones:** The process of rendering hormones inactive and causing them to be eliminated through the bile or urine occurs via the liver. Since estrogens and androgens are both growth hormones which stimulate cell division, elevation of their levels in the blood due to the liver's failure to remove them efficiently can cause their accumulation in

tissues. This in turn may lead to abnormal growths such as uterine fibroids, ovarian cysts, endometriosis, breast cysts and breast cancer, prostate enlargement or prostate cancer.

7. **Regulates cholesterol levels:** The liver rids the body of excess cholesterol, subsequently lowering the levels of low-density lipoproteins (LDL) cholesterol and triglycerides.

The body functions which are affected by emotional and mental activities are regulated by the liver. When the liver's blood storage and regulatory functions are affected and bleeding or clots result, the liver is usually in a diseased condition. The joints can become stiff and muscles can become spasmodic and numb when the liver blood is deficient as nourishment to the tendons and blood vessels is decreased. Conditions such as stroke, dizziness, headaches, tinnitus, deafness, fainting or convulsions can result due to severe liver blood deficiency. When the liver blood is so deficient that it cannot nourish the eyes, night blindness or blurring may result. Stress and negative or unhappy feelings can greatly affect the liver and cause a noticeable decline in liver vitality which can result in hiccups, hernia and pain surrounding the liver. The bowels may then also become constipated and sleep may become disturbed as nightmares or insomnia can occur.

Symptoms of a poorly functioning liver may include:
- Low energy
- Indigestion, bloating, constipation, gas or diarrhea
- Foggy thinking
- Weight gain
- Stiff, aching, weak muscles—especially lower back and shoulders
- Altered cholesterol levels
- Blood sugar abnormalities
- Sleep disturbances
- Easy bruising
- Brittle bones

- Fluid retention
- Kidney problems
- Slow wound healing

The liver plays a major role in the detoxification of numerous substances in the body whether they come from the environment, food or within the body (from hormones and other substances). In order to metabolize and eliminate these potentially harmful toxins, the liver has developed an intricate, two-step detoxification system. Together, these two phases convert toxins into water-soluble molecules that can be excreted from the body in the stool and urine.

Phase I Liver Detoxification System:

The Phase I detoxification system, composed mainly of the cytochrome P450 supergene family of enzymes, is generally the first enzymatic defense against foreign compounds. Most pharmaceuticals are metabolized through Phase I biotransformation. In a typical Phase I reaction, a cytochrome P450 enzyme (CypP450) uses oxygen and, as a cofactor, NADH, to add a reactive group such as a hydroxyl radical. As a consequence of this step in detoxification, reactive molecules which may be more toxic than the parent molecule are produced. If these reactive molecules are not further metabolized by Phase II conjugation, they may cause damage to proteins RNA and DNA within the cells. Several studies have shown evidence of associations between induced Phase I and/or decreased Phase II activities and an increased risk of disease such as cancer, systemic lupus erythematous and Parkinson's disease. Compromised Phase I and/or Phase II activity has also been implicated in adverse drug responses. This process is often referred to as bioactivation. In order to prevent bioactivation from occurring, there must be an orchestrated balance between Phase I and Phase II detoxification. Enhancements of both phases can be achieved through natural medicinal agents. Prior to this process, simple testing can be done in order to reveal the state of detoxification phases. For example, a quantity of caffeine is ingested and saliva samples are taken twice at specified intervals. The efficiency of caffeine clearance is directly related to the efficiency of Phase I detoxification. Rapid clearance shows enzyme induction either from xenobiotic exposure or toxins within the body. Slower rates indicate that CypP450 activity in the liver is abnormal. Patients with slower caffeine clearance will have more difficulty eliminating xenobiotics and other toxins. [2]

The primary nutrients required during phase I detoxification include B vitamins, vitamin C, folic acid, copper, magnesium and zinc, antioxidants including glutathione, N-acetyl cysteine, lipoic acid and the branched-chain amino acids leucine, isoleucine and valine. Phase I detoxification is further enhanced by indole-3-carbinol which is found in cruciferous vegetables such as broccoli, Brussels sprouts, cabbage and cauliflower. It is also enhanced by flavonoids including Silymarin from milk thistle, curcumin from the spice turmeric and polyphenol antioxidants from grape seeds and green tea. Nutrients required to support phase II detoxification include vitamins B5, B6, B12, and C, folic acid, selenium, zinc, molybdenum, glutathione and the amino acids glycine, cysteine, methionine, taurine and glutamine.

Phase II Liver Detoxification System:

One of the consequences of Phase I activation is that the product called the reactive intermediate is quite often more reactive—and potentially more toxic—than the parent molecule. Therefore, it is important that this molecule be converted to a non-toxic, water-soluble molecule as soon as possible. Conjugation of the reactive intermediate to a water-soluble molecule is accomplished by the Phase II conjugation reactions which include glucuronidation, sulfation, glutathione conjugation, amino acid conjugation, methylation and acetylation. These reactions require the water-soluble molecule that will be attached to the toxicant such as sulfate in the case of sulfation or glucuronic acid in the case of glucuronidation. They also use a large amount of energy in the form of adenosine triphosphate (ATP). In addition to energy repletion, Phase II reactions require an adequate, continually replenished amount of cofactors since these cofactors are attached to the toxins and then excreted. Several nutrients and phytonutrients support Phase

---

[2] Jacqueline Krohn and Frances Taylor, *Natural Detoxification: A Practical Encyclopedia*, revised edition, Hartley & Marks Publishers, 2000-01.

II reactions[3] including antioxidants, vitamins, amino acids and other substances the liver needs to have in ample supply to detoxify efficiently.

How a Stressed Liver Contributes to Weight Gain

Many people are unaware of the daily consumption of toxins that invade our bodies through our food supply. Specifically, refined carbohydrates, hydrogenated and processed vegetable oils, sugars, pesticides, packaged and processed foods all cause the liver to work overtime. The liver filters all of these poisons and automatically empties them into the gallbladder. The function of the gall bladder is to store and secrete bile in order to assist in the digestion of fats in the small intestine. If the toxin burden is too high in the gallbladder, bile cannot be expelled as it becomes congested due to increasing thickness. This results in further liver congestion. At this point the intestines, which normally use bile for breaking down fats, end up storing fat because the liver and bile flow are hindered. This cycle of impaired fat metabolism continues and results in increasing fat accumulation.

Once the liver is overburdened, a cascade of unfortunate events can lead to the formation of type 2 diabetes. In fact, having a fatty liver elevates the risk for type 2 diabetes by 500 percent![4] Carbohydrate sensitivity and resulting weight gain occur as sugar is converted to fat in the liver due to insulin resistance. This resistance arises from excess leptin production in fat tissues. Leptin is a hormone that is responsible for signaling the brain when the stomach is full. As leptin rises, its companion hormone, adiponectin, is decreased causing the insulin resistance. Insulin resistance develops over time as the cells in the body become desensitized to the effects of insulin. More and more insulin is needed to control blood sugar levels as the cells fail to recognize the previously familiar insulin due to overconsumption of sugar.

---

[3] Deann J. Liska, Ph.D. *ANSR–APPLIED NUTRITIONAL SCIENCE REPORTS,* 650 8/02 Rev. 8/05, "The Role of Detoxification in the Prevention of Chronic Degenerative Diseases"

[4] http://www.wellnessresources.com/studies/carbohydrate_restriction_improves_fatty_liver/

The cascade continues to spiral down as triglycerides or blood fats are elevated due to a congested liver which results in more weight gain. There are many factors that can perpetuate this process such as consuming excess calories between meals, late night snacking or over eating at meal time which all overwhelm the liver. In addition, inactivity of the body prevents the liver from sending much needed fuel to the muscles which then overwhelms the body with unburned excess fat and sugar. As the body is continually poisoned with excess toxic calories and inactivity, the very basis for which our metabolism was designed is incessantly brutalized!

Detoxification Questionnaire[5]

Signs and symptoms of liver toxicity are diverse. In order to determine if your liver is showing signs of stress, the following questionnaire will help to clarify your need for detoxification.

Point Scale

0- Never or almost never have the symptom

1- Occasionally have it, effect is not severe

2- Occasionally have it, effect is severe

3- Frequently have it, effect is not severe

4- Frequently have it, effect is severe

Head	Skin	Weight
Headaches	Acne	Binge or compulsive eating/drinking
Dizziness	Hives, rashes, dry skin	Craving certain foods
Insomnia	Hair loss	Excessive weight/Underweight
Faintness	Flushing, hot flashes, excessive sweating	Water retention
Total	Total	Total

---

[5] FLT Tools/Metagenics/Detox Questionnaire

The Ultimate Metabolic Plan©

Eyes	Heart	Energy/Activity
Watery or Itchy eyes	Chest pain	Fatigue, sluggishness
Swollen, reddened or sticky eyelids	Irregular or skipped heart beat	Apathy, lethargy
Bags or dark circles under eyes	Rapid heart beat	Hyperactivity
Blurred or tunnel vision	Pounding heart beat	Restlessness
Total	Total	Total
Ears	**Lungs**	**Emotions**
Itchy ears	Chest congestion	Mood swings
Ear aches, ear infections	Asthma, bronchitis	Anxiety, fear, nervousness
Drainage from ear	Shortness of breath	Anger, irritability, aggressiveness
Ringing in ears, hearing loss	Difficulty breathing	Depression
Total	Total	Total
Nose	**Digestive Tract**	**Mind**
Stuffy nose	Nausea, vomiting	Poor memory
Sinus problems	Diarrhea, constipation	Confusion, poor comprehension
Hay fever	Bloating, gas, belching	Difficulty making decisions
Sneezing attacks	Heartburn	Stuttering, slurred speech
Excessive mucous formation	Intestinal/Stomach pain	Poor physical coordination
		Learning disability
		Poor concentration
Total	Total	Total
Mouth/Throat	**Joints/Muscle**	**Other**
Chronic coughing	Pain, aches in joints	Frequent illness
Gagging, throat clearing	Arthritis	Frequent or urgent urination
Sore throat, hoarseness, loss of voice	Stiffness or limitation of movement	Genital itch or discharge
Swollen or discolored tongue, gums, lips	Feeling of weakness or tiredness	
Canker sores	Pain or aches in muscles	
Total	Total	Total

Total _____

Interpretation:

Above 50- **High**   15-49- **Moderate**   Below 14- **Low**

The Pathway to Optimal Liver Health

Fortunately through proper detoxification and targeted nutrient therapy, the liver can be fully restored back to optimal health. Initial healing of the liver begins with avoiding ongoing exposure to toxic foods

Foods to Detoxify the Liver

Nutrition is an essential component of the detoxification process as outlined in the following chart:

FOODS TO INCLUDE	FOODS TO AVOID
FRUIT TO INCLUDE: strawberries, citrus (except grapefruit), pineapple, apples, apricot, avocado, banana, blueberries, cherries, grapes, kiwi, mango, melons, nectarine, papaya, pear, peach, plums, prunes and raspberries Organically grown is always preferred.	**FRUIT TO AVOID:** grapefruit (grapefruit can alter detoxification enzyme function for up to 72 hours), all sweetened fruits (either canned or frozen) and sweetened fruit juice
VEGETABLES TO INCLUDE: arugula, asparagus, artichokes, bean sprouts, beets, bell peppers, bok choy, broccoli, Brussels sprouts, cauliflower, celery, cucumber, cabbage, eggplant, endive, escarole, all types of greens and lettuce, green beans, jicama, mushrooms, okra, green peas, radishes, spinach, squash (summer and winter), sweet potatoes, taro, turnips, yams and zucchini All vegetables should be fresh, raw, steamed, grilled, sautéed, roasted or juiced. Organically grown is always preferred.	**VEGETABLES TO AVOID:** corn (95% of the world's crop is genetically modified)
GRAINS TO INCLUDE: rice (brown, sushi, wild), potatoes, oats (gluten-free), quinoa, millet, tapioca, amaranth and buckwheat	**GRAINS TO AVOID:** corn and all gluten-containing products including wheat, spelt, kamut, barley and rye

LEGUMES TO INCLUDE: all legumes including peas and lentils (except soybeans)	**LEGUMES TO AVOID:** soybeans, tofu, tempeh, soy milk, soy sauce, and any product containing soy proteins
NUTS/SEEDS TO INCLUDE: all nuts except peanuts — almonds, cashews, macadamia, walnuts, pumpkin seeds, brazil nuts, and sunflower seeds — whole and raw or as a nut butter	**NUTS/SEEDS TO AVOID:** peanuts, peanut butter and peanut oil
MEAT AND FISH TO INCLUDE: all fresh or frozen wild fish (except shellfish) such as salmon, halibut, sole, mahi mahi, cod and snapper organic, hormone-free chicken, turkey, lamb and wild game (venison, buffalo, elk etc.)	**MEAT AND FISH TO AVOID:** tuna, swordfish, shellfish, beef, pork, cold cuts, hot dogs, sausage and canned meats
DAIRY AND EGGS TO INCLUDE: milk substitutes such as unsweetened coconut milk, rice milk, oat milk, hemp milk and almond or other nut milks	**DAIRY AND EGGS TO AVOID:** milk, cheese, cottage cheese, cream, butter, yogurt, ice cream, non-dairy creamers, soy milk and eggs
FATS TO INCLUDE: cold pressed oils such as olive, flaxseed, sesame, Grapeseed, red palm oil, walnut, hazelnut, pumpkin seed and coconut oil	**FATS TO AVOID:** margarine, butter, shortening, any processed or hydrogenated oils, peanut oil, vegetable oils, mayonnaise and fried foods
BEVERAGES TO INCLUDE: filtered or distilled water, green tea, herbal tea, pure fruit and vegetable juices, mineral water and roasted grain coffee substitutes	**BEVERAGES TO AVOID:** sodas and soft drinks (including sugar-free), alcoholic beverages, coffee, tea, or any other caffeinated beverages and sweetened fruit juice
SWEETENERS TO INCLUDE: green leaf stevia, blackstrap molasses, Luo Han fruit, pure maple syrup and xylitol	**SWEETENERS TO AVOID** white or brown sugar, high fructose corn syrup, honey, corn syrup, sucrose, dextrose, turbinado, nutritive corn sweetener and any artificial sweeteners, colors or flavors
HERBS/SPICES/CONDIMENTS TO INCLUDE: vinegars (except grain source), wasabi, mustard, horseradish, pesto (cheese-free), Himalayan sea salt and all herbs and spices	**HERBS/SPICES/CONDIMENTS TO AVOID:** salt, chocolate, ketchup, relish, soy sauce, BBQ sauce, chutney, MSG, BHA, BHT, nitrates, nitrites and any other chemical additive or preservatives

Liver cleansing is essential and central to healing the metabolism. Detoxifying the liver can be done on a regular basis and in more advanced cases, as part of an intensive detoxification program. There are many herbs that have the ability to detoxify the liver through their hepato protective and hepato restorative functions.

Herbs to Detoxify the Liver

Milk thistle *(Carduus marianus)*

Silymarin, a flavanolignan, is the main active compound that gives milk thistle its well-researched liver protecting effects. Silymarin protects the liver from damage by inhibiting damaging substances in the liver. Silymarin has the added ability to increase glutathione, one of the most critical nutrients for liver detoxification, in the liver, intestine and stomach.[6] There are hundreds of studies that involve the ability of milk thistle to protect and regenerate the liver. Milk thistle is proved to be useful in all liver conditions such as hepatitis, cirrhosis, liver damage, cholestasis and fatty liver. Silymarin's ability to promote the regeneration of damaged hepatocytes renders it as one of the most potent liver detoxifiers.

Turmeric *(Curcuma longa)*

Curcumin, one of the active compounds in turmeric, is a potent liver detoxifier and anti-inflammatory agent. Curcumin is of exponential use in Phase 2 detoxification pathways in the liver as it increases the levels of the enzymes needed to facilitate the action of Phase 2 detoxification. Curcumin also increases the production of bile from the liver which helps to expel toxins and reduce liver inflammation.

Burdock Root *(Arctium lappa)*

Burdock root is one of the foremost cleansing herbs, providing nourishing support for the blood, liver and natural defense system. It is rich in vitamins B1, B6, B-2, and E, plus manganese, copper, iron, zinc and sulfur. Burdock root contains inulin along with bitter compounds and mucilage which provides its ability to control liver damage and protection from further burdens to the

---

[6] Julieta Criollo, DNM, CHT, *Medicinal Herbs Quick Reference Guide,* 109.

liver. Burdock root also promotes the flow and release of bile which not only helps in cleansing the liver but also aids in the digestive process.[7]

Dandelion Root *(Taraxacum officinalis)*

The root of the dandelion plant is effective as a detoxifying agent, acting especially on the liver and gallbladder to remove toxins and waste products. It stimulates and tonifies the digestive system. Its cholagogue, or bile secreting effect, creates a mild laxative effect which allows for expulsion of toxins. Dandelion root is therefore useful in the treatment of liver conditions such as jaundice, metabolic toxicity, hepatitis and cholelithiasis (gallstones) as seen in two studies cited in *The Australian Journal of Medicinal Herbalism*.[8] Dandelion root has also been proven useful in the treatment of chronic conditions of the digestive system, conditions of the skin such as acne and eczema as well as joint problems such as arthritis.

Globe Artichoke *(Cynara scolymus)*

Globe artichoke contains a powerful compound called cynaropicrin which is a sesquiterpene lactone that stimulates the flow of bile from the liver and makes it a useful liver detoxifier and protector. Due to its ability to promote detoxification and improve bile flow, globe artichoke is useful in all cases of insufficient liver production and digestive insufficiency.

Blue Flag *(Iris versicolor)*

Blue flag has the ability to detoxify almost all channels of elimination. It stimulates the flow and release of bile from the liver, purges the intestines and promotes secretions from the pancreas. Blue flag also cleanses the blood of impurities and stimulates the lymphatic system which enhances whole body cleansing effects.

---

[7] The 4-Week Ultimate Body Detox Plan Michelle Schoffro Cook, DNM, DAc, CNC pg. 237

[8] The 4-Week Ultimate Body Detox Plan Michelle Schoffro Cook, DNM, DAc, CNC pg. 237

Yellow Dock *(Rumex crispus)*

The major plant chemicals in yellow dock are tannins, oxalates and anthraquinone glycosides (about 3-4%). Yellow dock also includes nepodin as well as other chemicals based on chrysophanol, physcion and emodin. These constituents produce alterative, gentle purgative, mild laxative and mild astringent tonic effects. The iron content of yellow dock makes it useful in treating anemia symptoms. Chrysarobin in yellow dock is found to relieve a congested liver.

The anthraquinone glycosides contained in yellow dock have a laxative effect on the bowels as well as on the liver and blood, making it beneficial in all detoxification strategies. The release of toxins from the tissues can create an increasingly symptomatic effect on the body if the channels of elimination are not working efficiently.

Barberry *(Berberis vulgaris)*

Barberry is a bark known for containing berberine, the powerful agent which has numerous actions including potent anti-microbial, hepato-protectant, bile secreting and liver detoxifying benefits. The bark contains a large number of alkaloids (berberine, berbamine, and oxyacantha) and tannins. Barberry is also effective in reducing nausea and vomiting, toning and strengthening the body and stimulating bowel action.

Nutrients to Detoxify the Liver

Liver detoxification processes can be facilitated with specific nutrients that have lipotropic actions. The function of a lipotropic nutrient is to aid in the flow of fat from the liver or gallbladder. In times of liver distress, it is essential to assist the process of detoxification until the liver is fully recovered and functioning normally. Nutrients that have antioxidant or protective actions such as Vitamin D, Alpha lipoic acid, Milk thistle (Silymarin), Vitamin E (tocotrienols) and N-acetyl-cysteine (NAC) are beneficial during times of liver toxicity or a fatty liver.

Alpha Lipoic Acid (ALA)

ALA is the remarkable "universal antioxidant" as it is both water and fat soluble, proving to have antioxidant effects on the inside and outside of the cells. ALA helps to neutralize the effects of all free radicals and enhances the antioxidant functions of vitamins C and E and glutathione.

Research shows that ALA is effective in neutralizing toxins from over-the-counter and prescription drugs before they can cause liver damage.

Calcium D-Glucarate

Calcium D-glucarate is a substance produced naturally in small amounts by humans. Supplementation of calcium D-glucarate has been shown to prevent recycling of hormones and environmental toxins, promoting liver detoxification and excretion of these potentially detrimental substances.

Glucuronidation is the normal process in the liver of attaching a glucuronic acid molecule to substances for detoxification and elimination from the body.* During phase II liver detoxification, toxic chemicals, steroid hormones and other fat-soluble toxins undergo glucuronidation and are then excreted through the bile or urine* Calcium D-glucarate helps assure this elimination process occurs uninterrupted.

Glutathione

Glutathione is one of the molecules used in Phase 2 detoxification and is produced in the body by the liver. Levels of glutathione naturally decrease with the aging process. Glutathione is made up of cysteine, glutamic acid and glycine. The amount of cysteine in the body will determine how much glutathione is produced. Glutathione has tremendous liver protecting effects which block the effects of environmental pollution, medications, radiation, mercury and other heavy metals. Glutathione aids in detoxification by removing fungicides, herbicides, carbamate, organophosphates, pesticides, nitrates, notrosamines, flavorings, plastics, steroids, phenolic compounds and certain medications from the liver.

Vitamin C

Vitamin C is a water-soluble antioxidant vitamin which is not produced within the body and therefore must be replenished through dietary means on a daily basis. Deficiencies in vitamin C have been shown to decrease the metabolism of xenobiotics by lowering the level of cytochrome P450.[9] Vitamin C aids in detoxification by combating all free radicals. Vitamin C also prevents damage from exposure to numerous hepato-toxic agents including pollutants, carbon monoxide, heavy metals, sulfur dioxide, carcinogens, stored lipophilic chemicals, medications, anesthetics, radiation, bacterial toxins and poisons.

N-Acetyl Cysteine (NAC)

NAC is thought to be an intermediate compound in cysteine metabolism which makes it a derivative of cysteine. NAC has the ability to boost glutathione levels which is critical to Phase 2 detoxification. NAC protects the liver from toxic compounds, has tremendous chemo-protectant effects and protects the body from radiation. NAC is a potent liver vasodilator which increases the blood flow to the liver, thereby enhancing its detoxification abilities.

Methionine

Due to methionine's sulfur content, it is a powerful antioxidant that has the ability to inactivate free radicals, support liver detoxification, protect cell membranes against lipid peroxidation and protect precious glutathione levels in the body. When levels of methionine in the body are sufficient, it has the added effect of preventing the accumulation of fat in the liver.

Coenzyme Q_{10} (COQ_{10})

COQ_{10} is the most powerful antioxidant in the body. COQ_{10}, also called ubiquinone, is a potent free radical scavenger which protects the cellular membranes against damage caused by toxins and is a crucial co-factor for energy production within the body.

---

[9] Jaqueline Krohn, MD and Frances Taylor, MA, *Natural Detoxification: A Practical Encyclopedia*, 276.

Vitamin B5

Vitamin B5, also known as pantothenic acid, is part of the B-complex family of vitamins. B5 is the main vitamin that is used in times of stress as it stimulates adrenal hormone production and supports adrenal function, preventing adrenal exhaustion during prolonged stress. B5 is a critical nutrient involved in Phase 1 detoxification, aiding the body by protecting against harmful radiation. It also counters the effects and toxicity of antibiotics, aids in the production of hydrochloric acid in the stomach and stimulates the synthesis of cholesterol.

Vitamin B6

Vitamin B6, also known as pyridoxine, is involved in more bodily processes than any other single nutrient and has an effect on both physical and mental health. B6 is needed for the metabolism of methionine, aids in the transport of amino acids across the cellular membrane and supports liver detoxification. B6 is also needed for the proper metabolism and use of protein, fats, carbohydrates and hormones.

Folic acid

Folic acid plays a role in both the Phase 1 and Phase 2 detoxification pathways. It is needed for the utilization of amino acids and is involved in protein metabolism as well as the production of RNA and DNA. Folic acid is required for the formation of both red and white blood cells.

Selenium

Selenium is an essential trace mineral that is found in glutathione peroxidase which is necessary for the recycling of glutathione. Considered to be one of the beneficial antioxidants, selenium protects the cellular membranes and prevents the breakdown of DNA. It also neutralizes free radicals and enhances the functions of vitamin C and E.

Zinc

Zinc is a trace mineral that is found in over ninety essential enzymes in the body.[10] Zinc is directly involved in Phase 1 detoxification as it is also found in alcohol dehydrogenase, an enzyme that detoxifies aldehydes. In addition, zinc supports liver detoxification and protects the liver from the toxic effects of chemicals. It is a component of superoxide dismutase and it reduces lipid peroxidation.

---

[10] Jaqueline Krohn, MD and Frances Taylor, MA, *Natural Detoxification: A Practical Encyclopedia,* 284.

Action Steps for Optimal Liver Health

1. Start the day with ½ lemon squeezed into 1 cup of warm water.
2. Consume half your body weight in ounces of filtered water daily.
3. Increase fiber consumption to 35 grams per day to assist in the elimination of fat soluble toxins. Choose high fiber foods such as ground flax seeds, psyllium, apple pectin, rice bran, beet fiber, oat fiber, chia seeds and sun fiber.
4. Consume liver cleansing foods such as beets, bitter greens, apples, lemons, garlic, onions, cabbage, broccoli, Brussels sprouts, kale, collards and cauliflower.
5. Use liver cleansing herbs such as Dandelion root, Artichoke, Milk thistle, Burdock root and Turmeric.
6. Detox the liver with Alpha lipoic acid, Calcium D-Glucarate, NAC, Selenium, Choline and Methionine.
7. Drink liver detoxifying tea with dandelion root, nettle root, red clover, licorice root, burdock root and cleavers.
8. Support the digestion with probiotics and digestive enzymes.
9. Avoid toxic foods such as sugar, processed foods, refined carbohydrates, pesticides, hydrogenated fats and artificial sugars.
10. Avoid smoking, alcohol, caffeine, pop and energy drinks.
11. Exercise regularly.

Stress and the Adrenals

In this day and age, stress levels have reached an all-time high. People are facing continual stress from the demands of our faced paced lifestyle and our adrenal glands are relentlessly preparing for disaster. The adrenal glands are responsible for governing our stress response by secreting hormones in order for us to respond to the stressors. When the adrenal glands are overworked, fat and calories are stored, energy is conserved and weight accumulates as our bodies prepare for adversity.

Stress can be defined as any perceived physical or psychological change that disrupts an organism's metabolic balance.[11] A chain of events is automatically activated in response to the stress. Signals are sent throughout the body through the communication efforts of the neuro-endocrine system, resulting in "fight or flight" responses. Some of these signals cause positive changes in order for the body to respond to the immediate or acute stress. Long-term or chronic stress poses too many challenges which overload the circuits and cause the systems of the body to eventually shut down.

As the adrenals continue to battle the daily on-going stressors, appetite greatly increases as the body craves extra fuel and stores this as fat around the abdomen, commonly referred to as "belly fat". The brain sends a message to the adrenals to release cortisol as our blood sugar levels drop and we begin to feel hungry. Our body is fueled with energy until we eat as cortisol

---

[11] *ANSR–APPLIED NUTRITIONAL SCIENCE REPORTS,* "Nutritional Management of Stress-Induced Dysfunction," YEAR.

activates glucose, fats and amino acids to maintain balance. When stress becomes chronic both insulin and cortisol remain elevated in the blood and the extra glucose is stored as fat–mostly in the abdomen.

It is now well documented that the abdominal fat cells have more receptors for cortisol than any other cells of the body. It was previously thought that abdominal fat was inactive tissue. Now scientists have discovered that belly fat is actually an active tissue which acts as an endocrine organ that responds to the stress response by welcoming more fat to be deposited.

Surveys and research reports conducted over the past two decades reveal that 43% of all adults suffer adverse effects due to stress. In fact, 75% to 90% of all visits to primary care physicians are in some way related to the adverse impact of psychosocial stress. Furthermore, an estimated one million workers are absent on an average workday because of stress-related complaints. The market for stress management programs, products and services has skyrocketed in the past decade and is estimated to currently exceed eleven billion dollars annually in North America.[12] While all age groups are affected by stress, the aging population faces compounded susceptibility to stress-induced disorders because of the accumulation of problems mediated by chronic, long-term stress.[13]

This means that at some point all of us have succumbed to the effects of stress in our lives in one way or another. Stress can have a way of creeping into our lives and slowly suffocating us. From symptoms such as chronic tension headaches to digestive upset and everything in between, we learn to live with the subtle effects of stress and they slowly become our "new normal".

It is not "JUST" stress! The following is a list of common physical symptoms that can arise from chronic and acute stress:

---

[12] *The American Institute of Stress*, "America's #1 health problem and job stress," November 2001. http://www.stress.org/problem.htm.

[13] W.A. Pedersen, R. Wan, and M.P. Mattson, *Mech Ageing Dev*, "Impact of aging on stress-responsive neuroendocrine systems," 2001;122(9):963-83.

- Depression and/or anxiety
- Increased abdominal fat
- Tired for no reason throughout the day but especially around 3pm
- Trouble getting up in the morning even when you go to bed at a reasonable hour
- Feeling rundown or overwhelmed
- Memory issues
- Difficulty concentrating or brain fog
- Lowered immune system
- Increased startle response
- Food cravings (salt and/or sugar)
- Blood sugar imbalances-Hypoglycemia

The General Adaptation Syndrome

Dr. Hans Selye, through his research on the physiological effects of chronic stress on rats developed the General Adaptation Syndrome (GAS). The General Adaptation Syndrome provides a summary of the physiological changes that follow stress. Dr. Selye observed three sets of responses whenever he injected rats with a toxin:

1. Adrenal gland enlargement
2. Lymph node decrease
3. Development of severely bleeding ulcers in the stomach and intestines

Over several years, Dr. Selye theorized that the same physiological changes take place in the human body in reaction to any kind of stress. These patterns had a tendency to result in disease conditions such as ulcers, arthritis, hypertension, arteriosclerosis and diabetes in humans. Dr.

Selye called the pattern the General Adaptation Syndrome. For decades, researchers have studied the syndrome and Dr. Selye's theories have held up to all levels of scientific scrutiny.

The three stages of the General Adaptation Syndrome include:
1. **Alarm Stage:** In the alarm stage, bursts of the hormones cortisol and adrenaline are released in response to a stressor, resulting in the traditional "fight or flight" responses.
2. **Resistance Stage:** In the resistance stage, the body uses high cortisol levels to free up stored energy to help the body physically resist the stressor. It is now known that a prolonged resistance stage may increase the risk of developing stress-related diseases. If cortisol levels remain elevated, symptoms may include feeling tired but wired, having difficulty sleeping, weight gain around the waist, high blood pressure, hair loss, muscle mass loss, and anxiety. Excess cortisol also interferes with the action of other hormones like progesterone, testosterone, and thyroid hormones which further creates more imbalances and increases symptoms.
3. **Exhaustion Stage:** At this stage, the adrenals are either depleted from producing too much cortisol or are reacting to the detrimental effects of high cortisol. This reduces the cortisol production significantly. Symptoms of low cortisol include fatigue (especially morning fatigue), increased susceptibility to infections, decreased recovery from exercise, allergies, low blood sugar, a burned out feeling, depression and low sex drive.

Chronic stress-induced dysfunction can create a significant loss of vitality and can result in serious long-term health problems. While stress is an inevitable consequence of modern life, the devastating damage caused by chronic stress cannot be ignored. A healthy diet, regular exercise, lifestyle changes, relaxation and holistic therapies can help to normalize the parameters of the stress response.

The first documented account of adrenal fatigue was in the 1800s in the medical textbooks, listing it as a clinical condition. Throughout early history, it was one of the most prevalent conditions commonly affecting the majority of adults. Conventional physicians were not kept abreast regarding the seriousness of adrenal fatigue despite the fact that there were very effective diagnostic tools and treatment protocols available. Over the past fifty years, adrenal fatigue has very seldom been diagnosed by conventional practitioners and has often been dismissed and treated with antidepressants along with the recommendation to "relax." Treatments such as these can cause the condition to progress into a complete demise of health for the patient as the natural progression of this pathology takes its course. Even today, adrenal fatigue is not an acknowledged medical condition by mainstream physicians although some forward-thinking doctors are now recognizing not only the prevalence but also the significance of this condition.

The adrenal glands are comprised of two small glands which are each the size of a large grape located on top of the kidneys. The main function of the adrenal glands is to provide stress coping and survival responses. Each adrenal gland is made up of two parts or cortices. The inner medulla modulates the sympathetic nervous system through secretion and regulation of two hormones called epinephrine (adrenalin) and norepinephrine (noradrenalin) which are responsible for the "fight or flight" response. The outer adrenal cortex comprises 80% of the adrenal gland and is responsible for producing over fifty different types of hormones in three major classes – mineralocorticoids, androgens and glucocorticoids. The main glucocorticoid hormone is cortisol which is produced in response to stress and is considered to be the primary "stress hormone" in the body. Cortisol is a life-sustaining adrenal hormone essential to the maintenance of homeostasis. It influences, regulates or modulates many of the changes that occur in the body in response to stress, including, but not limited to:

- Blood sugar (glucose) levels
- Fat, protein and carbohydrate metabolism to maintain blood glucose (gluconeogenesis)
- Immune responses
- Anti-inflammatory actions
- Blood pressure

- Heart and blood vessel tone and contraction
- Central nervous system activation

Higher and more prolonged levels of circulating cortisol (like those associated with chronic stress) have been shown to have negative effects, such as:[14]

- Impaired cognitive performance
- Dampened thyroid function
- Blood sugar imbalances such as hyperglycemia
- Decreased bone density
- Sleep disruption
- Decreased muscle mass
- Elevated blood pressure
- Lowered immune function
- Slow wound healing
- Increased abdominal fat which has a stronger correlation to certain health problems than fat deposited in other areas of the body. Some of the health problems associated with increased stomach fat are heart attacks, strokes, higher levels of "bad" cholesterol (LDL) and lower levels of "good" cholesterol (HDL) which can lead to other health problems.

Chronically lower levels of circulating cortisol (as in adrenal fatigue) have been associated with negative effects such as:

- Brain fog and mild depression
- Low thyroid function
- Blood sugar imbalances such as hypoglycemia
- Fatigue—especially in the morning and mid-afternoon
- Sleep disruption

---

[14] http://www.adrenalfatigue.org/cortisol-and-adrenal-function.html

- Low blood pressure
- Lowered immune function
- Inflammation

Symptoms Associated with Adrenal Fatigue:
- Always feeling cold
- Anxiety; fearfulness
- Chronic low-grade infections
- Frequent influenza
- Decreased sex drive
- Night sweats
- Needing to go to the bathroom at night
- Depression
- Environmental sensitivities
- Fibromyalgia
- Arthritis
- Headaches
- Hypoglycemia
- Inability to focus or concentrate
- Increased allergies
- Insomnia
- Light-headedness
- Lower back pain in kidney area and sacrum
- Low blood pressure
- Muscular weakness
- Poor memory
- Scanty perspiration

- Sensitivity to light, noise, touch and movement
- Feeling of exhaustion
- Weight gain or loss
- Feeling overwhelmed by little things
- Nausea
- Lightheaded when rising, lack of energy in the mornings and in the afternoons between 3:00 p.m. and 5:00 p.m.
- Feeling better suddenly for a brief period after a meal
- Often feeling tired from 9:00 p.m. to 10:00 p.m. but resisting going to bed
- Needing coffee or stimulants to get going in the morning
- Cravings for salty, fatty and high protein food such as meat and cheese
- For women: increased symptoms of PMS; periods are heavy and then stop or are almost stopped on the fourth day, only to start flowing again on the fifth or sixth day
- Pain in the upper back or neck for no apparent reason
- Feeling better when stress is relieved such as on a vacation
- Difficulty getting up in the morning

Causes of Adrenal Fatigue

In western society, chronic stress is very common and seemingly accepted as "normal." The most common causes of chronic stress are work pressure, career change, death of a loved one, moving homes, illness, and marital disruption. Adrenal fatigue occurs when the amount of stress overextends the capacity of the body to compensate and recover.

Stressors that can lead to Adrenal Fatigue include:[15]

- Anger
- Chronic fatigue
- Chronic illness
- Chronic infection—A commonly overlooked cause of adrenal fatigue is chronic or severe infection that gives rise to an inflammatory response. Such infection can occur sub-clinically with no obvious signs at all. Parasitic and bacterial infections including Giardia and H. pylori are often the main causes.
- Chronic pain
- Depression
- Fear and guilt
- Gluten intolerance
- Low blood sugar
- Mal-absorption
- Mal-digestion
- Toxic exposure
- Severe or chronic stress
- Surgery
- Working late hours
- Sleep deprivation
- Excessive exercise
- Excessive sugar in diet
- Excessive caffeine intake from coffee and tea
- Chronically infected root canal

---

[15] Adrenal Fatigue By: Michael Lam, MD, MPH www.DrLam.com

The following questionnaire is a key diagnostic tool used to evaluate the involvement of adrenal gland function in any disease state and is also used to aid in the diagnosis of adrenal fatigue. The questionnaire should be used in conjunction with specific laboratory testing to determine a definitive diagnosis of adrenal fatigue.

Adrenal Health Questionnaire[16]

Read each statement and decide its degree of severity based on the severity ranking system below.

0= Never
1= Occasionally (1-4 times per month)
2= Moderate in severity and occurs moderately frequently (1-4 times per week)
3= Intense in severity and occurs frequently (more than 4 times per week)

1. I get dizzy or see spots when standing up rapidly from a sitting or lying position.
2. I urinate more frequently than others and may need to get up at night.
3. I feel as though I might faint or black out.
4. I have chronic fatigue.
5. I have mitral valve prolapse or get heart palpitations.
6. I often have to force myself in order to keep going.
7. I have difficulty getting up in the morning.
8. I have low energy before the noon meal -approximately 11:00 a.m.
9. I have low energy in the late afternoon between 3:00 p.m. and 5:00 p.m.
10. I usually feel better after 6:00 p.m.
11. I often feel best late at night because I get a "second wind."
12. I have trouble getting to sleep.

---

[16] Fundamentals of Naturopathic Endocrinology Michael Friedman, MD pg. 218-220

13. I tend to wake early (approximately 3:00 a.m. to 5:00 a.m.) and have trouble getting back to sleep.
14. I have vague feelings of being generally unwell for no apparent reason.
15. I get swelling in the extremities such as the ankles.
16. I need to rest after times of mental, physical or emotional stress.
17. I feel more tired after exercise or being physical either soon after or the next day.
18. My muscles feel weak and heavy more that I think they should.
19. I have chronic tenderness in my back area near the bottom of my rib cage.
20. I have a weak back and/or weak knees.
21. I have restless extremities.
22. I am allergic to many things, such as foods, animals and pollens.
23. My allergies are getting worse.
24. I get bags or dark circles under my eyes which may be worse in the morning.
25. I have multiple chemical sensitivities.
26. I have asthma or get regular bouts of bronchitis, pneumonia or other respiratory infections.
27. I have dermatographism (a white line appears on my skin if I run my fingernail over it and the line persists for one minute).
28. I have an area of pale skin around my lips.
29. The skin on the palms of my hands and soles of my feet tend to be red/orange in color.
30. I tend to have dry skin.
31. I tend to get headaches and a sore neck and shoulders.
32. I am sensitive to bright light.
33. I frequently feel colder than others around me.
34. I have decreased tolerance to cold.
35. I have Raynaud's syndrome (extremely cold hands/feet).
36. My temperature tends to be below normal when measured with a thermometer.
37. My temperature tends to fluctuate during the day.

38. I have low blood pressure.

39. I become hungry, confused or shaky if I miss a meal.

40. I crave sugar, sweets or desserts.

41. I use stimulants such as tea or coffee to get started in the morning.

42. I crave food high in fat and feel better with high-fat foods.

43. I need caffeine (chocolate, tea, coffee, colas) to get me through the day.

44. I often crave salt and/or foods high in salt such as potato chips.

45. I feel worse if I eat sweets and no protein for breakfast.

46. I do not eat regular meals.

47. I eat fast food often.

48. I am sensitive to pharmaceutical or nutritional supplements.

49. I have taken steroid medications for a long term or at a high dose.

50. I have symptoms that improve after I eat.

51. I tend to be thin and find it difficult to put weight on.

52. I have feelings of hopelessness and despair or have been diagnosed with depression.

53. I lack motivation because I do not feel I have the energy to get things done.

54. I have decreased tolerance toward other people and tend to get irritated by them.

55. I get more than two colds per year.

56. It takes me a long time to recover from illness.

57. I get rashes, dermatitis, eczema, psoriasis or other skin conditions.

58. I have an autoimmune disease.

59. I have fibromyalgia.

60. I have had mononucleosis or been diagnosed with Epstein Barr virus.

61. I do not exercise regularly.

62. I have a history of large amounts of stress in my life.

63. I tend to be perfectionist.

64. My health is negatively affected by stress.

65. I tend to avoid stressful situations for the sake of my health.
66. I am less productive at work that I used to be.
67. My ability to focus mentally is generally impaired.
68. Stressful situations hinder my ability to focus.
69. Stress causes me to become overly anxious.
70. I startle easily.
71. It can take me days or weeks to recover from a stressful event.
72. I tend to get digestive disturbances when tense.
73. I tend to get unexplained fears and phobias.
74. My sex drive is very low or non-existent.
75. My relationships at work and or home tend to be strained.
76. My life contains insufficient time for fun and enjoyable activities.
77. I have little control over my life and I feel "stuck."
78. I tend to get addicted easily to drugs, alcohol or foods.
79. I suffer from post-traumatic distress disorder.
80. I have or have had an eating disorder.
81. I have gum disease and/or tooth infections or abscesses.
82. I have symptoms of premenstrual syndrome (PMS)- *for women only*
83. My periods are irregular and/or affected by stress- *for women only*

Interpretation:

Total score:

    Under 40: very slight or no adrenal fatigue

    41-80: mild adrenal fatigue

    81-120: moderate adrenal fatigue

    Above 120: severe adrenal fatigue

The following are three additional tests that can be performed in order to further determine the function or lack of function of the adrenal glands:

ADRENAL FUNCTION TEST #1-Postural Hypotension:

Postural hypotension (also known as orthostatic hypotension) is a drop in blood pressure that occurs upon rising from a horizontal position. It is commonly expressed as a feeling of dizziness or lightheadedness, a "head rush," or "standing up too fast."

To do this test, a blood pressure cuff is required. Lie down and rest for five minutes. Take a blood pressure reading while still horizontal. Then stand up and take another reading.

Normally, a healthy blood pressure reading should rise ten to twenty points. If it drops, particularly by ten points or more, hypoadrenia is indicated. Generally, the bigger the drop, the greater the adrenal insufficiency.

ADRENAL FUNCTION TEST #2-Iris Contraction Test

For this test, a weak flashlight or penlight and a mirror are both needed. In a dark bathroom or closet, wait a minute for the eyes to adjust to the dark. This will allow the pupils to dilate (open) fully. Then, shine the flashlight into the eyes and watch the reaction of the pupils for at least thirty seconds.

The light should cause the iris to contract, making the pupils (the dark spot in the center of your eye) smaller. Normally, they should stay that way but if adrenal gland fatigue is occurring, the iris will be weak and will not be able to hold the contraction. It will either waver between being contracted and relaxed or will contract initially but then open up after ten to thirty seconds.

As with the postural hypotension test, the degree to which you "fail" this test is an indicator of the degree of adrenal insufficiency you are experiencing.

ADRENAL FUNCTION TEST #3-Sergent's Adrenal White Line

With the fingernail or the dull end of a spoon, draw a line across the belly. In moderate to severe cases of adrenal fatigue, the line will stay white and even get wider over the course of time. The "normal" reaction would be for the line to almost immediately turn red.

This test has historically been used to indicate severe adrenal fatigue and Addison's disease. Milder cases of adrenal fatigue may not exhibit this sign.

Adrenal Stress Index Salivary Testing

The panel utilizes four saliva samples. Salivary cortisol measurement reflects the free (bioactive) fraction of serum cortisol. The test report shows the awake diurnal cortisol rhythm generated in response to real-life stress.

The cortisol/DHEA relationship highlights the many facets of stress maladaptation. The cortisol/DHEA ratio helps determine the projected time for recovery and the substances (hormones, supplements, botanicals) that promote this recovery. The cortisol/DHEA ratio regulates a multitude of functions.

The panel measures P17-OH levels in order to evaluate the efficiency of the conversion of adrenal precursors into cortisol. Certain adrenal fatigue patients who are genetically predisposed to low production of cortisol will not benefit from exogenous supplementation of pregnenolone or progesterone.

The panel includes fasting and non-fasting insulin measurements. The insulin values are used to diagnose insulin resistance-functional insulin deficit (pre-diabetes) as well as to correlate elevated cortisol with insulin to help explain glycemic dysregulation problems.

Interpretation of The Adrenal Stress Index Test for DHEA and Cortisol Levels[17]

Levels of DHEA and cortisol vary according to the level of stress and for how long that stress has been occurring. Increasing cortisol production is the normal response to stress and is highly desirable so long as the stress is removed and the adrenal glands can recover.

Ongoing, unremitting stress means the adrenal gland and the whole body is in a constant state of alert and does not get time to recover and eventually functionally fails. Therefore, there are several stages of adrenal function gradually leading to failure:

1. **Normal levels of cortisol and normal levels of DHEA.** Normal result, indicating a normal adrenal gland.
2. **High levels of cortisol and normal levels of DHEA.** This indicates a normal short-term response to stress.
3. **High levels of cortisol and high levels of DHEA.** The adrenal gland is functioning normally but the patient is chronically stressed. If the stress is removed, the adrenal gland will recover completely.
4. **High levels of cortisol and low levels of DHEA.** The body cannot make enough DHEA to balance the cortisol. This is the first sign of adrenal exhaustion and the first abnormal response to chronic stress. The patient needs a long break from whatever that chronic stress may be. The most common chronic stress is hypoglycemia but the stress could also be caused by insomnia or mental, physical or emotional overload. DHEA can be supplemented to make the patient feel better but it must be part of a package of recovery without which worsening can be expected.
5. **Low levels of cortisol and low levels of DHEA.** The gland is so exhausted that it can't make cortisol or DHEA. By this time, patients are usually severely fatigued.

---

[17] http://www.prohealth.com/ME-CFS/library/showArticle.cfm?libid=14383&B1=EM031109C

6. **Low levels of cortisol and borderline or normal levels of DHEA.** This probably represents the gland beginning to recover after a long rest. DHEA may be used to help patients feel better while they continue their program of rest and rehabilitation.

Restoring the Adrenals

Adrenal function can be completely restored with the proper treatment plan. Eliminating and reducing external stressors is the key to complete healing. Balance can be achieved by encompassing a combination of nutritional therapy, herbal medicine and targeted nutrients for adrenal restoration coupled with stress management.

Nutritional Guidelines for Optimizing Adrenal Health

Nutritional Factors Affecting Adrenal Fatigue

During adrenal fatigue, the cells of the body respond to stress by speeding up cellular metabolism and subsequently burning precious nutrients at a much higher pace. Very quickly the cells use up much of the body's supply of stored nutrients and deficiencies may ensue, further exacerbating the issues. Nutrition becomes a critical part of the healing and a diet abundant in good quality food is crucial. In addition, not only is the quality of the food important but also the timing in which it is consumed. The adrenal hormone cortisol aids in maintaining balanced blood sugar levels to meet the body's constant demand for energy. During adrenal fatigue, cortisol levels drop lower than normal, making it very difficult to maintain balanced blood sugar levels. As a result, hypoglycemia (low blood sugar) often accompanies adrenal fatigue.

Eating Patterns
- Do not let more than 3 hours go between meals.
- It is crucial to eat before 10:00 a.m. to replenish glycogen (stored blood sugar) levels.

- Eat lunch early, between 11:00 a.m. and 11:30 a.m., as the body quickly uses up the nutrients from the morning meal.
- Have a nutritious snack between 2:00 p.m. and 3:00 p.m. in order to prevent the typical hypoglycemic tendencies that occur between 3:00 p.m. and 4:00 p.m.
- Dinner should be eaten between 5:00 p.m. and 6:00 p.m.
- Just before bed, a small snack may be required to prevent panic attacks, sleep disturbances and anxiety reactions throughout the night.

Foods to Consume
- Combine a fat, protein and carbohydrate at every meal and snack.
- Eat 15-20 grams of protein at each meal (2-3 eggs or 6-8oz of animal protein).
- Eat 5 cups of brightly colored vegetables each day.
- Limit fruit to 2 servings per day and avoid tropical fruits due to their high sugar content. Combine protein with fruit to slow the release of sugar into the bloodstream (nuts, nut butter and organic plain yogurt).
- Eliminate or minimize grains- avoid grain based foods at breakfast and lunch.
- Celtic sea salt can be added to foods in moderation to improve adrenal function.
- Add one to two tablespoons of essential oils into grains, vegetables, and proteins daily.

Foods to Avoid
- Refined sugar including cakes, pies, doughnuts, cookies and other foods containing white flour, sugar and chocolate.
- All dairy except for organic, plain yogurt.
- Stimulating beverages such as coffee, colas, black tea, hot chocolate and energy drinks.
- Avoid alcohol.
- Eating fruit in the morning (the naturally-occurring fructose in the fruit will cause a spike in blood sugar and an eventual drop which is exacerbated in the morning).

- Processed foods that rob the cells of the body of the critical energy needed to heal. In addition, processed foods put extra stress on the liver which is often already sluggish in adrenal fatigue.

The Impact of Gluten on Adrenal Fatigue

Many people that are suffering with adrenal fatigue have hidden gluten sensitivities. Gluten is extremely stressful to the body and further depletes the adrenals when consumed. One of the most important aspects to healing from adrenal fatigue is to eliminate gluten completely. Gluten sensitivities do not always cause digestive symptoms, in fact there is more evidence of damage to the nervous system than there is to the digestive system when it comes to gluten. Sensitivity symptoms can include:

- Weight gain
- Inflammation, swelling or pain in your joints such as fingers, knees or hips
- Mood issues such as anxiety, depression, mood swings, schizophrenia and ADD
- Digestive issues such as gas, bloating, cramping, diarrhea and even constipation
- Keratosis Pilaris also known as "chicken skin" on the back of your arms
- Eczema, acne, rashes and other skin conditions
- Fatigue, brain fog or lack of concentration
- Neurologic symptoms such as dizziness, vertigo and peripheral neuropathy
- Hormone imbalances such as PMS, PCOS or unexplained infertility
- Migraines and chronic headaches
- Autoimmune disease such as Hashimoto's thyroiditis, Rheumatoid arthritis, Ulcerative colitis, Lupus, Psoriasis, Scleroderma or Multiple sclerosis

Herbal Medicine Indicated for Adrenal Fatigue

There is a class of herbs known as "adaptogens." A herb classified as an adaptogen has the unique ability to aid in the body's response system to stress. These herbs allow the body to better adapt to stress and provide a buffering or balancing action that counteracts an exaggerated adrenal response to stress. Adaptogens affect both the adrenal gland function directly as well as the HPA axis (Hypothalamus-pituitary-adrenal axis). There are six main herbs that fall into this category:

Licorice Root (*Glycyrrhiza glabra*)

Licorice is one of the most well-known adaptogenic herbs with use dating back thousands of years.[18] The action of licorice comes from the triterpenes, glycyrrhizin and its aglycone component, glycyrrhetinic acid. The triterpenes are metabolized to a similar structure as the adrenal cortical hormones which may be responsible for licorice root's anti-inflammatory action. Glycerrhizin inhibits liver damage and increases antibody production through a stimulation of interleukin.[19] Glycyrrhetinic acid has been shown to be similar in structure to corticosteroids and therefore have adrenocortico mimetic actions. Research has shown that licorice can increase cortisol levels and help to resolve issues with low blood pressure. Through its effects on the kidneys, it also improves the body's ability to retain sodium and magnesium and subsequently reduces issues with frequent urination.

There has been much research on the concern that licorice can increase blood pressure. This is due to the fact that licorice blocks the conversion of cortisol into cortisone which can produce higher amounts of circulating cortisol. Most patients with adrenal fatigue typically have low blood pressure but simple monitoring of blood pressures levels will allow for the successful and safe administration of licorice root.

---

[18] Fundamentals of Naturopathic Endocrinology Michael Friedman, MD pg. 127

[19] Fundamentals of Naturopathic Endocrinology Michael Friedman, MD pg 127

Ashwagandha Root (*Withania somnifera*)

Ashwagandha is an ancient Indian herb with therapeutic actions dating back to at least 1000 BC. Ashwagandha is commonly called Indian ginseng although it is not related to any species of ginseng, it does, however, have similar therapeutic effects. Traditionally, ashwagandha has been prescribed in the healing of a wide variety of illnesses and has been well established as a tonic for restoring strength and vigor. Research has shown that ashwagandha can influence hormone activity by providing support to the HPA axis function. As an adaptogen, it also aids in the adaptability to both physical and chemical stress by increasing catecholamine production.[20] More than thirty-five active constituents have been identified in ashwagandha but it is the alkaloids and steroidal lactones that are responsible for many of its effects.

Ashwagandha studies have shown that the plant protects against the physical ravages of stress, preventing adrenal mass increase and vitamin C depletion. In addition, stress-induced increases of both blood urea nitrogen and lactic acid are avoided.[21]

Rhodiola (*Rhodiola rosea/Rhodiola crenulata*)

Rhodiola comes from the mountainous regions of Siberia. It is thought to strengthen the nervous system, fight depression, enhance immunity, elevate the capacity for exercise, enhance memory, aid weight reduction, increase sexual function and improve energy levels. It has long been known as a potent adaptogen. Since rhodiola administration appears to impact central monoamine levels, it might also provide benefits and be the adaptogen of choice in clinical conditions characterized by an imbalance of central nervous system monoamines.

There have also been claims that this plant has great utility as a therapy in asthenic conditions (decline in work performance, sleep disturbances, poor appetite, irritability, hypertension, headaches and fatigue), developing subsequent to intense physical or intellectual strain, influenza and other viral exposures as well as other illness. Two randomized, double-blind, placebo-controlled

---

[20] Archana R Namasivayam A. Antistressor effect of Withania somnifera. J Ethnopharmacol 1998 Oct; 62 (3): 209-14

[21] Archana R Namasivayam A. Antistressor effect of Withania somnifera. J Ethnopharmacol 1998 Oct; 62 (3): 91-93

trials of the standardized extract of rhodiola root provide a degree of support for these claimed adaptogenic properties.[22]

Siberian Ginseng Root (*Eleutherococcus senticosus*)

Siberian ginseng first became medically recognized for its therapeutic benefits in the 1950s and 1960s when Dr. Brekham studied the attributes of this herb. Eleutherosides have been found to be the main active constituent in Siberian ginseng. Beta-sitosterol which possesses anti-cancer, anti-inflammatory and anti-hyperglycemic properties is the other active constituent. In addition, the lignans that are produced in this herb are responsible for its immunostimulating effects. The eleutherosides were found to have specific binding affinity for adrenal receptor sites including glucorticoid, mineralcorticoid and progestin receptors. Siberian ginseng is typically useful in states of exhaustion as it is considered to be one of the more stimulating adaptogens and is also useful in depression and debility.

Siberian ginseng has a wide range of therapeutic benefits including rejuvenating adrenal function, increasing resistance to all forms of stress, normalizing metabolism, regulating neurotransmitters and counteracting mental fatigue.

Schisandra (*Schisandra chinensis*)

Schisandra has been traditionally used to promote energy and alleviate exhaustion and immune system disturbances caused by stress. Schisandra has also been taken to strengthen the sex organs and promote mental function. The herb counteracts testosterone-induced atrophy of the adrenal glands in animal studies. Ingestion of the fruit of Schisandra has been shown to increase adrenal and spleen function in animals.

As many as thirty lignans have been identified in Schisandra that are responsible for increasing metabolism of deoxycholic acid which is a risk factor for hepatocarcinogenesis. For this reason, Schisandra is used in cases of poor liver function, hepatitis and liver cancer. Due to the fact that it

---

[22] http://www.herbwisdom.com/herb-rhodiola.html

increases the secretion of sexual fluids in both males and females, it is useful in cases of low libido. In addition, Schisandra balances fluid and relieves urinary frequency as it tones and strengthens kidney function. It is also useful in cases of excessive thirst and night sweats and in cases of insomnia as it acts to calm the body. Mental illness, memory lapse and irritability also improve significantly with the use of Schisandra. It is considered to be a deep immune activator.

Relora

Relora is a proprietary blend of the plant extracts from the Magnolia and Phellodendron plants and has been used with dramatic results for anxiety and anxiety related eating. Relora comprises at least two compounds selected from magnolol, honokiol and magnoflorine and proprietary Phellodendron (amurense) extract. Prolonged secretion of cortisol in response to stress may have a negative impact on the body. Clinical research has shown that Relora may help decrease salivary cortisol levels and provide support for controlling irritability and emotional ups and downs.

Specific Nutrients in the Treatment of Adrenal Fatigue

Vitamin C

Vitamin C, also known as ascorbic acid, is the primary vitamin for adrenal gland function. With increasing levels of cortisol, the need for vitamin C rises. Vitamin C is critical to the manufacture of adrenal steroid hormones and the homeostasis of the adrenal hormone cascade. Vitamin C is used along the entire adrenal pathway and has antioxidant functions within the adrenal cortex.

Naturally occurring vitamin C always occurs with bioflavonoids. The addition of bioflavonoids to supplemental ascorbic acid more than doubles the effectiveness of the vitamin C. Bioflavonoids are essential if ascorbic acid is to be fully metabolized and utilized by the cells of the body. The best found ratio is one to two bioflavonoids to ascorbic acid.

Vitamin C is a water-soluble vitamin and is utilized and excreted by the body very quickly. Therefore, doses should be administered several times throughout the day. Individual dosing needs can be determined through a bowel tolerance functional test. Start by taking 1000mg of vitamin C (this should include 500mg of bioflavonoids) and continue this dose every hour until bowel movements become watery. Decrease the dose by 1000mg and continue with that level each day in divided doses.

Vitamin B Complex

As coenzymes, the B vitamins are essential components in most major metabolic reactions. They play an important role in energy production including the metabolism of lipids, carbohydrates and proteins. B vitamins are also important for blood cells, hormones, adrenal glands and nervous system function. As water-soluble substances, B vitamins are not generally stored in the body in any appreciable amounts (with the exception of vitamin B-12). Therefore, the body needs an adequate supply of B vitamins on a daily basis. Dosage: 100 mg-200mg per day with food

Vitamin B5 (Pantothenic Acid)

Vitamin B5 is essential for healthy adrenal and immune function. In particular, B5 serves as the starting material for the synthesis of coenzyme A which acts as the carrier of acyl groups in oxidation, acetylation and decarboxylation reactions. It is also instrumental in the synthesis of fatty acids and adrenal hormones. Thus, B5 is important for energy production as acetyl CoA is converted from B5 and is crucial for the conversion of glucose into energy. Dosage: 500mg-1500mg per day with food

Vitamin B6 (Pyridoxine HCl)

Vitamin B6 and its bioactive form, pyridoxal 5'-phosphate (P5P), are essential for such processes as amino acid metabolism, neurotransmitter synthesis and glycogen breakdown. Vitamin B6 is a co-factor in several of the enzymatic pathways in the adrenal cascade. It is also involved in heme synthesis, conversion of tryptophan to niacin and proper metabolism of fatty acids. Due to the fact that the conversion of pyridoxine to P5P occurs in the liver, a compromise in liver function can have deleterious effects on P5P levels in the body, placing one at risk of vitamin B6 deficiency. Recollection of dreams often significantly improves when vitamin B6 deficiency levels are corrected. Dosage: 50-100mg per day with food

Magnesium

Adequate magnesium is critical to adrenal gland fatigue recovery. Magnesium is essential to the production of enzymes and the energy necessary for the adrenal hormonal pathway. Magnesium is a mineral that functions as a coenzyme for nerve and muscle function. It is essential for the formation of bones, regulation of body temperature, energy metabolism as well as DNA and RNA synthesis. The need for magnesium increases during periods of heightened stress because it is a cofactor for several regulatory enzymes, especially those involved with energy production and nervous system function. Clinical studies have shown that magnesium supplements decrease anxiety and chronic stress. Dosage: 400-600mg per day

Pregnenolone

Pregnenolone is the first hormone to be made from cholesterol in the adrenal pathway. It can be converted into several other adrenal hormones including DHEA, sex hormones, aldosterone and cortisol. In advanced cases of adrenal fatigue, it is often required to begin replacing chronically deficient adrenal hormones. Beginning with pregnenolone will allow the body the opportunity to determine which hormones the pregnenolone will be converted into based on specific needs. Often the body naturally converts the pregnenolone into sex hormones which are severely decreased in adrenal fatigue. A specific function of the sex hormones is to act as antioxidants and protect the body from the oxidative damage from high levels of circulating cortisol which is a key factor in rapid aging. Dosage: 20-30mg of the bioidentical cream per day

DHEA (Dehydroepiandrosterone)

DHEA levels often become depressed during adrenal fatigue. DHEA is one of the main androgen hormones secreted by the adrenal glands and is the precursor to many of the adrenal sex hormones. It is an important hormone base from which testosterone, progesterone and corticosterone, either directly or indirectly, can be derived. After age forty, the amount produced in the body starts to decline. Very little is left by age seventy. Research indicates that taking DHEA supplements may help to prevent cancer, arterial disease, multiple sclerosis and Alzheimer's disease. DHEA may even be useful in the treatment of lupus and osteoporosis, may help to improve memory and may enhance the activity of the immune system. DHEA should only be used in extreme cases, the patient should be closely monitored and levels should be tested regularly. Dosage: DHEA for chronic fatigue, 5-25 mg (only if testing shows that levels are low) helps with energy production and the effects of stress.

Adrenal Cell Extracts

The adrenal cell extracts restore, support and transform adrenal fatigue. They enhance adrenal activity and speed recovery. Adrenal cell extracts are not replacement hormones but rather contain the essential constituents for adrenal repair, including cellular contents such as the nucleic acids RNA and DNA. In addition, cell extracts contain concentrated nutrients in the form and proportion used by the adrenals to properly function and recover. They contain only minute amounts of the actual hormones in the adrenal gland. Dosage: varies depending on individual preparations

Phosphorylated Serine (PS)

PS is of extremely beneficial use in stage two adrenal dysfunction when cortisol levels are high. PS has the unique ability to decrease circulating cortisol and allow for a dramatic decrease in symptoms such as anxiety and insomnia. It is important to obtain lab testing to determine when to administer PS as it should be taken one hour before cortisol levels are elevated. Dosage: 500mg-1000mg one hour before elevated cortisol levels

Stress Management

De- Stressing your life is the most important step you can take on the road to optimal health. There will always be times of stress in our lives that we cannot control but there are also many areas of stress in our lives that we can control. The first step is to recognize your stress. Think about all the areas in your life that cause you stress- work, home life, relationships with family and friends, body image, finances and past issues to name a few. Take inventory of all the things that are affecting you and write a list of everything that comes to mind no matter how big and unavoidable or how small and insignificant. Write it ALL down! Take that list and objectively decide which things you can actually change and write an action step beside each one. Get to work and start eliminating and dealing with the stressors that you can and then the ones that you cannot change will feel much more manageable.

Find an outlet for your stress. We need to "spend" all of those excess stress hormones that are circulating our bodies. Find something that you love to do and feel good doing. Things such as exercise, dance, art, music and journaling are just a few examples of the ways that you can help yourself manage the effects of stress in your life.

Action Steps for Optimal Adrenal Health

1. Get tested- Salivary Adrenal testing will help to determine your level of adrenal fatigue.
2. Find an outlet for your stress (exercise, dance, art, music etc.).
3. Recognize your stress- learn to identify your stress before it consumes you.
4. List all of your stress and eliminate the stress that you can change.
5. Balance your blood sugar by eating every 3 hours.
6. Eliminate the top dietary stressors-gluten, sugar, alcohol, caffeine and dairy.
7. Get adequate rest, sleep and gentle exercise- walking, stretching, swimming etc.
8. Take adrenal restoring herbs like Licorice root, Ashwagandha, Relora, Rhodiola, Siberian ginseng and Schisandra.
9. Take supportive nutrients such as Vitamin B-complex, Vitamin C, Magnesium, Phosphorylated Serine (PS) and DHEA.
10. Take Adrenal cell Extracts to boost adrenal function.

The Thyroid Connection and Weight Gain

A dysfunctional thyroid can affect almost every aspect of your health. Imbalances of the thyroid are connected to many hormone issues. These can include breast cancer, uterine fibroids, ovarian cysts, endometriosis, infertility, postpartum depression, miscarriage, PMS, amenorrhea (no cycles) and menorrhagia (heavy cycles). Hypothyroidism or underactive thyroid is often linked with adrenal fatigue, estrogen dominance and progesterone deficiency. Thyroid dysfunction is one of the most under-diagnosed hormonal imbalances of aging, together with estrogen dominance and metabolic syndrome.

More than 13 million Americans have been diagnosed with thyroid disease and another 13 million people are estimated to have undiagnosed thyroid problems. About 10 percent of the adult population is afflicted with this frequently overlooked disease of epidemic proportions. Women are five times more likely to be diagnosed with hypothyroidism than men.

The thyroid is a butterfly-shaped gland in the neck below the Adam's apple. The thyroid is the master metabolizer and energy generator lever that fires up the genes that keep cells of the body properly functioning. Every cell in your body has thyroid hormone receptors and the thyroid is therefore fundamental in all aspects of health. The thyroid hormone, like other hormones, is regulated by an extensive negative feedback system. The system starts in the hypothalamus of the brain that releases thyrotropin-releasing hormone (TRH). TRH signals the pituitary gland to release thyroid stimulating hormone (TSH). TSH in turn instructs the thyroid gland to make thyroid hormones and release them into the bloodstream. When the level of thyroid hormones in your body is high, a negative feedback system exists to reduce the production of TSH, and vice-versa. Therefore, a high TSH is indicative of hypothyroidism, while a low TSH can be indicative of hyperthyroidism.[23]

The following illustration depicts the location of the thyroid gland:[24]

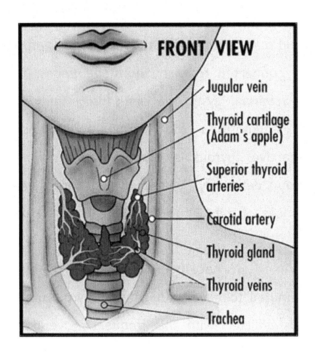

---

[23] Michael Lam, MD, MPH www.DrLam.com

[24] http://www.google.ca/images/thyroid gland

Symptoms of Thyroid Imbalance[25]

The following chart outlines the differences between an under functioning thyroid (hypothyroid) and an over functioning thyroid (hyperthyroid):

Hypothyroid State	Hyperthyroid State
General Symptoms	**General Symptoms**
A.M. underarm temperature lower than 97.8 F	A.M. underarm temperature higher than 98.2° F
Carpal tunnel syndrome, tendonitis, joint stiffness and swelling, muscle weakness, fibromyalgia, muscle and joint pain, increased rheumatoid arthritis	Fatigue and weakness
Puffy face, especially around the eyes, swelling of hands and feet, weight gain, difficulty losing weight	Weight loss, increased appetite
Slower speech, thick tongue, deep, hoarse voice	Hyperactive state, racing thoughts, nervousness
Feels cold all the time, hard to stay warm	Feels warm most of the time, intolerant to heat
Frequent or chronic infections, particularly fungal or viral	Osteoporosis, increased calcium loss in urine
Low DHEA, DHEA-S and pregnenolone	High DHEA-S and pregnenolone sulfate

Hypothyroid State	Hyperthyroid State
Reproductive System	**Reproductive System**
Low libido	Low or very high libido
PMS, prolonged heavy period, longer menstrual cycle	Irregular periods, usually more frequent, light menstrual flow
Failure to ovulate, infertility, easy miscarriage	Infertility
Premature delivery, stillbirth	
Production of breast milk when not nursing, elevated prolactin	
Decreased sex hormone binding globulin-means more available estrogen, estrogen dominance	Increased sex hormone binding globulin-means less available estrogen
Severe menopausal symptoms	Increased menopausal symptoms

---

[25] Complete Natural Medicine Guide to Women's Health Sat Dharam Kaur, ND pg. 417-18

Can have increased susceptibility to breast cancer and other cancers	Increased susceptibility to fibrocystic breast disease, breast cancer and other cancers

Hypothyroid State	Hyperthyroid State
Cardiovascular System	**Cardiovascular System**
Slow pulse (less than sixty beats per minute)	Fast pulse (more than one hundred beats per minute), heart palpitations
Low blood pressure	High blood pressure (systolic, shortness of breath)
Sleep apnea	Swollen, red, bulging eyes
High cholesterol, high LDL, and triglycerides, low HDL, macrocytic anemia	Reduced platelets causing easy bleeding
High homocysteine and lipoprotein (a)	Enlarged heart, angina, increased risk of heart disease, increased risk of mitral valve prolapse
	Palpable goiter (swelling) of thyroid gland in throat, atrial fibrillation (fluttering beats), arrhythmia

Hypothyroid State	Hyperthyroid State
Hair, Skin, and Nails	**Hair, Skin, and Nails**
Hair is dry, brittle, falling out, loss of lateral 1/3 of eyebrow	Hair loss, thinning, greasiness
Dry scaly skin, tendency to eczema, psoriasis, no perspiration	Increased perspiration, vitiligo (white patches)
Yellowing of the skin, especially on the palms	Raised thickened skin over shins
Thin brittle nails with transverse grooves	Soft nails, easily torn, clubbing of fingertips

Hypothyroid State	Hyperthyroid State
Nervous System	**Nervous System**
Mental-emotional symptoms	Mental-emotional symptoms
Fatigue and muscle weakness, anemia	Over activity, insomnia, eyes sensitive to light
Depression, memory loss, poor concentration	Confusion, disorganized thinking, depression
Slow thinking, emotional instability, agoraphobia, anxiety, irritability, apathy, dementia	Nervousness, anxiety, panic attacks, irritability, mood swings, paranoia, aggression, psychosis
Slow reflexes, particularly Achilles tendon reflex	Shakiness and tremor (especially in hands)
Frequent headaches	

Hypothyroid State	Hyperthyroid State
Gastrointestinal Tract	**Gastrointestinal Tract**
Constipation	Frequent bowel movements, diarrhea, increased thirst
Low stomach acid, mineral deficiencies-poor zinc absorption	Increased need for vitamins and minerals; zinc and calcium deficiency

Low thyroid function is a common and often overlooked or improperly diagnosed cause of unwanted weight gain.

The first step is to find out if you have any of the chronic symptoms of hypothyroidism or any of the diseases associated with hypothyroidism.

Ask yourself if you have any of the following symptoms:
- Weight gain or inability to lose weight
- Sluggishness in the morning
- Poor concentration and memory
- Low-grade depression
- Swollen feet/swollen eye lids
- Dry skin
- Hoarse voice
- Excessive ear wax
- Thinning hair
- Coarse hair
- Being very sensitive to cold and having cold hands and feet
- Low body temperature
- Muscle pain
- Weakness or cramps
- Low sex drive

- Fluid retention
- High cholesterol

Causes of Hypothyroidism

Thyroid function can slowly become out of balance or can suddenly become an issue. **The following list outlines the most common causes of low thyroid function:**

- High or low cortisol, low DHEA
- Estrogen dominance, HRT, BCP
- Progesterone deficiency
- Extreme hormonal fluctuations such as pregnancy, childbirth and menopause
- Increased or prolonged stress
- Sluggish liver
- Iron deficiency anemia
- Nutritional deficiencies (zinc, selenium copper, manganese, magnesium, Vitamins A, B2, B3, B6, B12, C and E
- Iodine deficiency
- Heavy metal toxicity (lead, cadmium and mercury interfere with the conversion of T4 into T3 in the liver)
- Injury to the cervical vertebrae
- Accumulating fluoride levels
- Radiation from x-rays
- Food allergies (gluten, animal protein and dairy)
- Candida overgrowth and bowel toxicity

Testing for Hypothyroidism

Standard laboratory tests have been established for thyroid disease although there are additional hormones that need to be evaluated when examining the many aspects of thyroid imbalances.

The Basal body Temperature test can be used as an indication to the presence of a thyroid disorder. Hormones secreted by the thyroid gland reflect the metabolic rate as the body temperature is examined. This is deemed as the most sensitive thyroid test.

Basal Body Temperature Test
1. Shake down the thermometer to below 95°F and place it by your bed before going to bed at night.
2. On waking, place the thermometer in the armpit for a full ten minutes. It is important to move as little as possible; lying and resting with closed eyes is best. Do not get up until the 10 minutes has passed.
3. After 10 minutes, read and record the temperature and date.
4. Record the temperature for at least three mornings at the same time of day.

    A normal temperature is 97.8-98.2°F or 36.6-36.8°C with fluctuations that occur with the menstrual cycle. Menstruating women must perform the test on the 2nd, 3rd and 4th days of the menstrual cycle.

Post-Menopausal women can perform the tests on any day. If your temperature is consistently lower than this, there may be an indication of hypothyroidism. If the temperature is consistently higher this may be an indication of hyperthyroidism.

Complete Thyroid Profile

A complete thyroid profile includes free T4, free T3, TSH and TPO (Thyroid Antibodies) and can indicate the presence of an imbalance in thyroid function. The presence of elevated thyroid antibodies can show up long before imbalances of other thyroid hormones and therefore testing for these is crucial in identifying thyroid imbalances. Discrepancies exist in the range for TSH. In Canada the range is 0.5- 5.5; however, in the USA the range is 0.5 -3.0. Many Integrated health practitioners agree that TSH should fall below 2.0 for optimal thyroid health. It is imperative that all thyroid hormones be evaluated before dismissing a diagnosis of low thyroid function and not just TSH which is most commonly the only hormone tested.

It is also highly advisable to also check estrogen, progesterone, testosterone, cortisol and DHEA levels as they are greatly affected by thyroid function. Alternatively imbalances in these hormones can also negatively affect the function on the thyroid. Adrenal function must be evaluated and optimized before treatment of low thyroid function is administered. Stimulating thyroid function in a co-existing case of adrenal fatigue can greatly increase thyroid symptoms. Therefore restoring adrenal function is a crucial part of thyroid restoration.

Dried Urine - Iodine

Iodine is an essential component of the thyroid hormones T4 and T3. About 90% of iodine consumed from any source (e.g., diet, supplements, medication) is eliminated in urine within twenty-four to forty-eight hours; therefore, urine is an excellent source to determine an individual's iodine status. When urine iodine levels are outside optimal ranges (too low or high), thyroid hormone synthesis can be abnormal. Therefore, information about urinary iodine status can provide clues to thyroid dysfunction and the means to correct it.

Optimizing Thyroid Function

Nutritional Factors Affecting Thyroid Disorders

1. Avoid gluten in the case of autoimmune hypothyroidism. Gluten will act as an inflammatory agent in the case of autoimmune hypothyroidism. Testing for celiac disease in this case is also recommended but regardless of the outcome of the testing, strict gluten avoidance is recommended.
2. Testing for the presence of food allergies and sensitivities is highly recommended in the case of elevated Thyroid antibodies. Eliminating allergens is one of the steps to reduce the immune system's attack on the thyroid gland.
3. Eat nutrient dense food, preferably organic (to avoid pesticides and other chemicals that place additional stress on the body) including plenty of fruits, vegetables and cold water fish.
4. If iodine deficiency is suspected, include kelp, organic/unprocessed sea salt in the diet.
5. Avoid processed and refined foods, especially sugar, white flour and foods containing a lot of additives (food dyes, flavoring such as MSG, food coloring and especially artificial additives).
6. Include food such as whole grains, green vegetables, lean meat, brown rice and other foods that are rich in B vitamins. Some B vitamins (B2, B3, and B6) are needed for production/conversion of thyroid hormones. They also help build resistance to stress and participate in productions of energy, cell proliferation and the metabolism of fats, proteins and carbohydrates.
7. Lima beans, tomatoes and salmon are high in potassium and vitamin B5. Potassium can help alleviate symptoms of excess adrenaline (avoid salt to support the sodium–potassium balance) and vitamin B5 (considered the anti-stress vitamin) helps with the functioning and production of the adrenal glands hormones.

8. If possible, buy organic products to reduce intake of pesticide residues and other chemicals and hormones in animal-foods.
9. Hypothyroidism: Eat sea vegetables such as kelp, dulse, nori, hiziki and wakami as a source of iodine.

Herbal Medicine Indicated for Hypothyroidism

Bladderwrack (*Fucus vesiculosos*)

Bladderwrack contains three main constituents- iodine, alginic acid and fucoidan. The iodine in Bladderwrack helps those people deficient in this trace mineral to regulate and improve thyroid function, thus it is beneficial for hypothyroidism and goiter. It works as an anti-inflammatory and possesses anti-rheumatic properties to relieve arthritis and rheumatism. Bladderwrack's anti-bacterial properties help ward off bacteria and viruses. The alginic acid constituent, a type of dietary fiber, is useful in relieving constipation, diarrhea and heartburn. The fucoidan constituent, another type of fiber, contributes to lowering cholesterol and glucose levels. The symptoms of iodine deficiency can be relieved with seaweed therapy (Bladderwrack) at five grams per day. It contains weak hormone activity with the compound diiodotyrosine which is the building block for T3 and T4 production.

Ashwagandha (*Withania somnifera*)

Ashwagandha (Withania somnifera) directly affects the production of thyroid hormones. Animal studies during the late 1990's demonstrated its ability to directly act on thyroid tissue to bring about a rise in serum levels of thyroid hormones. Serum levels of the thyroid hormones can also be raised in humans and so excessive dosages should be avoided. Studies have been conducted to investigate the effects of Ashwagandha on thyroid and liver function. Mice given high doses (1.4g/kg) of the root extract showed significant increases in serum levels of T3 and T4. Furthermore, the extract was shown to reduce hepatic lipid peroxidation significantly while increasing the activity of superoxide dismutase and catalase. These results indicate that Ashwagandha stimulates both thyroid and hepatic antioxidant activity. [26]

Coleus (*Coleus Forskohlii*)

Increased cellular cyclic AMP results in inhibition of platelet activation, decreased likelihood of blood clots, reduced release of histamine, decreased allergy symptoms, increased force of contraction of the heart, relaxation of the arteries and other smooth muscles, increased thyroid function, increased fat metabolism and increased energy along with possible weight loss. Cyclic AMP and the chemicals it activates comprise a second messenger system that is responsible for carrying out the complex and powerful effects of hormones in the body. Coleus (Coleus forskohlii) contains forskohlin which is specifically able to mimic the effect of TSH in thyroglobulin (TG) production and promote secretion of T3 and T4.

Guggul (*Commiphora mukul*)

Guggul (Commiphora mukul) is considered a rejuvenating herb and a stimulant in Ayurvedic medicine. The resin of the Commiphora mukul tree, termed "Guggul" or "guggulipid," has been associated with thyroid stimulating activity. Guggul causes the thyroid to increase iodine uptake and increase production of thyroid hormones. Studies in both animals and humans have shown that Guggul can also modulate cholesterol levels. [27]

Specific Nutrients in the Treatment of Thyroid Disorders

Iodine and Tyrosine

Iodine deficiency is well accepted as the most common cause of endocrinopathy (goiter and primary hypothyroidism). Iodine deficiency is most critical in pregnancy due to the consequences

---

[26] Kohrle J, Spanka M, Irmscher K, Heschrd. Flavanoid Effects on Transport Metabolism and Action of Thryoid Hormones. Prog. Clin. Biol. Res. 1988;280:323-40

[27] http://www.restorativemedicine.org/pages/hypothyroidism_moderate.html

for neurological damage during stages of fetal development and lactation. The safety of therapeutic doses of iodine above the established safe limit of 1.0 mg may be evident in the lack of obvious toxicity in the Japanese population that consumes twenty-five times the median intake of iodine consumption in the United States. The Japanese population suffers no demonstrable increased incidence of autoimmune thyroiditis or hypothyroidism. Studies using 3 to 6mg doses to effectively treat fibrocystic breast disease may reveal an important role for iodine in maintaining normal breast tissue architecture and function. Iodine may also have important antioxidant functions in breast tissue and other tissues that concentrate iodine via the sodium iodide symporter.

L-tyrosine is an amino acid necessary for the synthesis of thyroxine (T4) and triiodothyronine (T3). In the process of thyroid hormone synthesis, iodine binds to two positions on the tyrosyl ring of tyrosine. Thus, a deficiency of this important amino acid could contribute to low thyroid hormone levels. Studies have found that tyrosine may be beneficial for treating fatigue which is a common symptom of low thyroid activity. Iodine is necessary for the formation of T4 but appears to have no effect on peripheral conversion of T4 to T3. Goitrogenic foods can cause a relative iodine deficiency by binding to iodine, making it inaccessible for thyroid hormone synthesis.

Trace Minerals

All the essential minerals bound to citric acid including copper and iron are required for proper thyroid hormone balance. Besides providing a well-absorbed chelate, citric acid has potential health benefits of its own. As an important Krebs cycle intermediate, it is essential for metabolism in all living organisms. Citric acid has been shown to inhibit urinary precipitation of calcium oxalate and phosphate crystals, preventing the formation of kidney stones. Specifically, zinc (50mg per day) and selenium (200 mcg per day) are an essential part of the conversion of T4 into T3 occurring in the liver.

Vitamin C and the B vitamins riboflavin (B2), niacin (B3), and pyridoxine (B6) are also necessary for normal thyroid manufacture.

Armour Thyroid

Armour Thyroid is a natural, porcine-derived thyroid hormone replacement containing both T4 and T3. Armour thyroid is used in the treatment of hypothyroidism. Thyroid glands are collected from USDA-approved grain-fed pigs. The thyroids are processed, dried, powdered and compounded to produce Armour Thyroid tablets. Since the amount of thyroid hormone present in the thyroid gland may vary from animal to animal, the T4 and T3 are measured in both the raw material and in the actual tablets. This ensures that Armour Thyroid tablets are the same from tablet to tablet.

Action Steps for Optimal Thyroid Function

1. Get proper testing- TSH, Free T4, Free T3 and TPO.
2. Identify and eliminate hidden food allergies.
3. Eliminate gluten regardless of allergy due to its connection to autoimmune hypothyroidism.
4. Identify and eliminate heavy metals toxicity as it impairs the ability of T4 to convert to T3.
5. Restore nutritional deficiencies such as Zinc and Selenium as these are needed for T4 to T3 conversion.
6. Treat any underlying adrenal fatigue before engaging in thyroid treatments as it is crucial to have properly balanced cortisol for thyroid function.
7. Take nutrients to boost thyroid function-Tyrosine, Iodine, Copper, Selenium, Zinc, Vitamin A and Vitamin D3.
8. Take herbs to restore thyroid function such as Kelp, Ashwagandha, Guggul, Blue Iris, Nettles and Forskohlii.
9. Replace thyroid deficiency with Armour Thyroid- a natural desiccated thyroid hormone containing both T3 and T4 in combination.
10. Treat any other underlying hormone imbalance such as progesterone, estrogen and testosterone.

Estrogen Dominance

Up until their mid to late 30s, most women live in relative harmony with their hormones. The effects of subtle changes can begin to occur around the average age of 35. Like a dimmer switch slowly going down, women start to notice slight changes in their menstrual cycle as PMS can begin to last longer, moods become more unstable and the metabolism slows as the balance between estrogen and progesterone is tipped.

Somewhere around her early to mid-40s, when a woman enters into perimenopause, her progesterone levels begin to fluctuate and drop even more. Over time, as the progesterone is depleted, the balancing effects on estrogen is lost and the body goes into a state of "estrogen dominance" which causes weight gain, especially around the mid-section.

Dr. John Lee, the world's authority on natural hormone therapy, coined the phrase "estrogen dominance." This condition occurs when deficient, normal or excessive estrogen levels are not equally balanced with progesterone. Estrogen and progesterone work synergistically with each other to achieve and maintain hormonal balance in the body. The main cause of many hormonal issues is not the absolute deficiency of estrogen or progesterone but rather when estrogen dominates the hormonal pathway over progesterone.

Presently, the average female begins puberty at approximately age twelve. She seldom lactates, has few children and menstruates about 350 to 400 times during her lifetime. This frequent menstruation of the modern-day female has been associated with the increased occurrence of a variety of hormonal conditions, including infertility, cancer, fibroids, anemia, migraines, mood swings, abdominal pain, fluid retention and endometriosis. In stark contrast, one hundred years ago, the average female started her menses at approximately age sixteen. It was common to not only have more children but to conceive at a younger age. She therefore spent more time lactating and had fewer menstrual cycles. In total, women at that time experienced the menstrual cycle only about 100 to 200 times in their lifetimes.

From age thirty-five to fifty (perimenopause), there is a 75% reduction in production of progesterone in the body. Estrogen, during the same period, only declines about 35%. In North America, the prevalence of estrogen dominance syndrome approaches 50% in women over thirty-five years old. By menopause, the total amount of progesterone made is extremely low, while estrogen is still present in the body at about half its pre-menopausal level.

With the gradual drop in estrogen but severe drop in progesterone, there is insufficient progesterone to counteract the amount of estrogen in the body. According to Dr. John Lee, the key to hormonal health is achieving the balance of progesterone and estrogen. For optimum health, the progesterone to estrogen ratio should be approximately between two hundred and three hundred to one of progesterone to estrogen, meaning progesterone should be two hundred to three hundred times higher than estrogen.

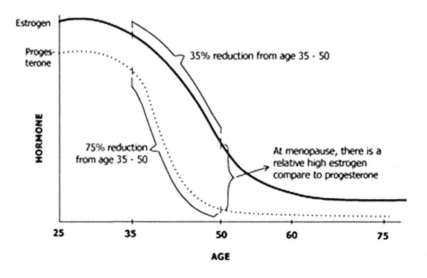

The symptoms and conditions associated with estrogen dominance are: [28]

- Acceleration of the aging process
- Allergies including asthma, hives, rashes and sinus congestion
- Autoimmune disorders such as lupus erythematosis and thyroiditis and possibly Sjoegren's disease
- Breast cancer
- Breast tenderness or fibrocystic breasts
- Cervical dysplasia
- Cold hands and feet as a symptom of thyroid dysfunction
- Copper excess
- Decreased sex drive
- Depression with anxiety, agitation or irritability
- Dry eyes
- Early onset of menstruation
- Endometrial (uterine) cancer
- Fat gain, especially around the abdomen, hips and thighs
- Fatigue
- Foggy thinking
- Gallbladder disease
- Hair Loss
- Headaches
- Hypoglycemia
- Increased blood clotting (increasing risk of stroke)
- Infertility
- Irregular menstrual periods
- Insomnia

---

[28] http://www.johnleemd.com/store/estrogen_dom.html

- Magnesium deficiency
- Memory loss
- Mood swings
- Osteoporosis
- Polycystic ovaries
- Premenopausal bone loss
- PMS
- Prostate cancer (men only)
- Sluggish metabolism
- Thyroid dysfunction mimicking hypothyroidism
- Uterine cancer
- Uterine fibroids
- Water retention, bloating
- Zinc deficiency

Causes of Estrogen Dominance

During a normal menstrual cycle, estrogen is the naturally dominant hormone for the first two weeks leading up to ovulation. In the last two weeks of the menstrual cycle, estrogen is naturally balanced by progesterone. As a woman enters perimenopause and begins to experience anovulatory cycles (cycles where no ovulation occurs), estrogen can often go unopposed, causing hormonal imbalance. Anovulatory cycles are, however, only one potential factor in estrogen dominance. In industrialized areas such as North America, there can be many other causes leading to estrogen dominance, including:

1. **Exposure to In Utero Xenoestrogens**: When symptoms of anovulation or progesterone deficiency are noted in puberty, exposure to xenoestrogens in utero can be a factor. Five

hundred thousand to eight hundred thousand follicles are created in the embryo, each enclosing an immature ovum when a female embryo develops in the womb. Outward changes to the pregnant mother may not be obvious when exposed to toxic estrogen-like chemicals. However, the fragile ovarian follicles are extremely sensitive to environmental pollutants which can be toxic. The fetus is therefore increasingly affected by environmental toxins which may then damage its ovarian follicles.

2. **Exposure to Petrochemical Compounds**: Petrochemical compounds are found in general consumer products such as creams, lotions, soaps, shampoos, perfumes, hair sprays and room deodorizers. These compounds have estrogen-like chemical structures and may have estrogen-mimicking effects. Other sources of xenoestrogens include car exhausts, petro chemically derived pesticides, herbicides and fungicides, solvents and adhesives such as those found in nail polish, paint removers, glues, dry-cleaning chemicals, practically all plastics and industrial waste such as PCBs and dioxins. Synthetic estrogens from urine of women taking HRT and birth control pills are flushed down the toilet and eventually find their way into the food chain and back into the body. They are fat-soluble and non-biodegradable.[29]

3. **Exposure to Industrial solvents**: Solvents are a family of chemicals that are often overlooked as a common source of xenoestrogens. These chemicals enter the body through the skin and accumulate quickly in the lipid-rich tissues such as myelin (nerve sheath) and adipose (fat). Some common organic solvents include alcohol such as methanol, acetaldehyde, glycol, ethylene glycol and acetone. They are commonly found in cosmetics, fingernail polish and fingernail polish remover, glues, paints, varnishes and other types of finishes, cleaning products, carpets, fiberboards and other processed woods. Pesticides and herbicides such as lawn and garden sprays as well as indoor insect sprays are also

---

[29] http://www.drlam.com/articles/Estrogen_Dominance.asp

sources of minute amounts of xenoestrogens. While the amount may be small in each, the additive effect from years of chronic exposure can lead to estrogen dominance.[30]

4. **Exposure to Hormone Replacement Therapy (HRT):** The hormones used in HRT are different in structure to the hormones naturally found in humans. This differing structure is processed in a lab in order to patent the medication and therefore make an economic profit. One of the most popular HRT drugs is called Premarin and has been the mainstay choice of doctors prescribing HRT. Premarin contains 48% estrone and only a very small amount of progesterone which is insufficient to have a significant opposing effect. The excessive estrogen from HRT can lead to an increased chance of DNA damage and can result in endometrial and breast cancer.

5. **Exposure to Xenoestrogens in Commercially Raised Cattle and Poultry:** Twenty-five million pounds per year, or half the antibiotics used in the United States each year, are used in livestock. These antibiotics enter our food supply and result in hormone disruption as we consume them as meat. In poultry farms, it now only takes six weeks to grow a chicken to full size, compared to four months in 1940. Feed containing a cocktail of hormone-disrupting toxins including pesticides, antibiotics and drugs is used to combat disease and is necessary due to the overcrowded conditions of animal warehouses.

6. **Exposure to Commercially Grown Fruits and Vegetables Containing Pesticides**: Over the years, but especially over the past 50 years, several billion pounds of pesticides have been released into the environment. These pesticides are similar in structure to estrogen and therefore can disrupt our hormonal system. Pesticides that were previously banned make their way back to our food supply illegally. Approximately five billion pounds of chemicals have been added to the world each year in the form of pesticides, herbicides, fungicides and other biocides. It is estimated that the average person eats seventy-five pounds of

---

[30] http://www.drlam.com/articles/Estrogen_Dominance.asp

illegal pesticides per year just by following the guidelines of eating five servings of fruits and vegetables a day if purchasing them from non-organic sources.[31]

7. **Overproduction of estrogen**. Excessive estrogen can arise from ovarian cysts or tumors.

8. **Stress.** The effects of chronic stress cause a reduction in progesterone levels and leads to adrenal gland exhaustion. This causes the hormonal pathway to favor estrogen over progesterone. The adrenal glands are further depleted as excessive estrogen causes insomnia and anxiety. The cycle continues as there is a further reduction in progesterone output and even more estrogen dominance results. After a few years in this vicious cycle, the adrenal glands become exhausted. This dysfunction leads to blood sugar imbalance, hormonal imbalances and chronic fatigue.

9. **Obesity.** Fat has an enzyme that converts adrenal steroids to estrogen. The higher the fat intake, the higher the conversion of fat to estrogen. Studies have shown that estrogen and progesterone levels fell in women who switched from a typical high-fat, refined-carbohydrate diet to a low-fat, high-fiber and plant-based diet even though they did not adjust their total calorie intake.

10. **Liver diseases**. Estrogen breakdown is reduced in individuals suffering from liver diseases such as cirrhosis from excessive alcohol intake. Estrogen levels increase in the body when the liver is unable to complete the detoxification process due to certain medical conditions, drugs or alcohol that can impair liver function.

11. **Deficiency of Vitamin B6 and Magnesium**. These are important constituents of hormonal balance and are necessary for the neutralization of estrogen in the liver. Too much estrogen also tends to create deficiencies of zinc, magnesium and B vitamins. Increased consumption of sugar, fast foods and processed foods results to a depletion of magnesium.

12. **Increase in caffeine consumption.** Caffeine intake from all sources has been linked to higher estrogen levels. This is true regardless of age, body mass index (BMI), caloric intake, smoking and alcohol habits. Studies have shown that women who consumed at least 500

---

[31] http://www.drlam.com/articles/Estrogen_Dominance.asp

mg of caffeine daily, the equivalent of four or five cups of coffee, had nearly 70% more estrogen during the early follicular phase than women who consumed no more than 100 mg of caffeine daily or less than one cup of coffee. Tea is not much better as it contains about half the amount of caffeine as coffee. The exception is herbal teas which contain no caffeine.

Diagnosing Estrogen Dominance

Do you have estrogen dominance (progesterone deficiency)?

This questionnaire lists symptoms and other factors most commonly found in women suffering from Estrogen Dominance and/or Progesterone Deficiency. Read each question carefully and see if it applies to you. The point value is listed. Add your score at the bottom of the page.

_____ Do you have premenstrual breast tenderness? 4 points
_____ Do you have premenstrual mood swings? 4 points
_____ Do you have premenstrual fluid retention and weight gain? 4 points
_____ Do you have premenstrual headaches? 4 points
_____ Do you have migraine headaches? 3 points
_____ Do you have severe menstrual cramps? 4 points
_____ Do you have heavy periods with clotting? 3 points
_____ Do you have irregular menstrual cycles? 3 points
_____ Do you have uterine fibroids? 3 points
_____ Do you have fibrocystic breast disease? 3 points
_____ Do you have endometriosis? 2 points
_____ Have you had problems with infertility? 2 points
_____ Have you had more than one miscarriage? 2 points
_____ Do you have joint pain? 1 point

_____ Do you have muscle pain? 1 point

_____ Do you have decreased libido? 3 points

_____ Do you have anxiety or panic attacks? 2 points

Total Score

< 5 It is not likely that you have estrogen dominance.

5-8 Possibility of estrogen dominance.

9-20 Estrogen dominance is probable.

> 20 Indicates that estrogen dominance is very likely.

The diagnosis of estrogen dominance can also be achieved through lab testing.

Estradiol and progesterone levels and their ratio are an index of estrogen/progesterone balance. An excess of estradiol, relative to progesterone, can explain many symptoms in reproductive age women.

Testosterone levels can also be either too high or too low. Testosterone in excess, often caused by ovarian cysts, leads to conditions such as excessive facial and body hair, acne, oily skin and hair. Polycystic ovarian syndrome (PCOS) is thought to be caused, in part, by insulin resistance. On the other hand, too little testosterone is often caused by excessive stress, medications, contraceptives and surgical removal of the ovaries. This leads to symptoms of androgen deficiency including loss of libido, thinning skin, vaginal dryness, loss of bone and muscle mass, depression and memory lapses.

Sex Hormone Binding Globulin (SHBG) binds tightly to circulating estradiol and testosterone, preventing their rapid metabolism and clearance. This limits their bioavailability to tissues. SHBG gives a good index which indicates the extent of the body's overall exposure to estrogens.

Restoring Estrogen Balance

Reduce Exposure to Xenoestrogens

The following is a list of tips for avoiding some of the most common xenoestrogens[32]:

- Avoid organochlorines which is one of the largest sources of xenoestrogens. They are used in pesticides, dry cleaning, bleaching of feminine-hygiene products and the manufacture of plastics.
- Avoid Bisphenol A, a breakdown of polycarbonate, which is used in many plastic bottles. It is found in the lining of many food cans and juice containers.
- Avoid heating plastics, plastic lined-items and polystyrene foam (e.g., Styrofoam) because the polycarbonates escape during the heating process.
- Use glass, ceramics or steel to store/consume foods and liquids.
- Choose organic produce, especially when buying thin-skinned fruits and vegetables.
- Buy hormone-free animal products (e.g., eggs, poultry, meats and dairy) to avoid xenoestrogen injections and bovine growth hormones that are added to non-organic animal products.
- Avoid butylated hydroxyanisole (BHS) which is a common food preservative found in processed food.
- Avoid non-organic coffee and tea.
- Use reverse-osmosis filtered water or purchase your own filter for drinking and bathing.
- Avoid parabens and stearalkonium chloride which are contained in many creams and cosmetics. Choose natural brands with preservatives made from minerals or grapefruit seed extract.
- Avoid parabens and phenoxyethanol which are 100% absorbed into the body. They are used in most skin lotions, creams, soaps, shampoos and cosmetics as preservatives.

---

[32] http://www.suite101.com/content/xenoestrogens-and-your-health-a205476.

- Avoid phthalates which are commonly found in baby lotions and powders.
- Avoid sunscreen containing benzophenone-3, homosalate, 4-methyl-benzylidene camphor, octal-methoxycinnamate or octal-dimethyl-PABA.
- Avoid artificially-scented perfumes, deodorizers and air fresheners which contain phthalates.
- Avoid petrochemical-based perfumes.
- Avoid nail polish and nail polish remover which contain harsh chemicals.
- The birth control pill contains high concentrations of synthetic estrogen. Choose a condom or diaphragm gels without surfactants. Use a non-spermicidal condom.
- Avoid hormone replacement therapy which contains synthetic estrogen. Instead, use a paraben-free progesterone cream.
- Dryer sheets, fabric softeners and detergents contain petrochemicals that can be absorbed by the skin. Use laundry detergent with fewer chemicals or use white vinegar and baking soda.
- Be aware of noxious gas that comes from copiers and printers, new carpets and fiberboards.
- Do not inhale and protect your skin from electrical oils, lubricants, adhesive paints, lacquers, solvents, oils, fuel, industrial wastes, packing materials, harsh cleaning products and fertilizers.
- Avoid pesticides, herbicides, fungicides, parathion, plant and fungal estrogens, industrial chemicals (cadmium, lead, mercury), conjugated estrogens/medroxyprogesterone (e.g., Prempro®, diethylstilbestrol (DES), Premarin, Cimetidine (e.g., Tagamet®), marijuana, insecticides (e.g., Dieldrin, DDT, Endosulfan, Heptachlor, Lindane/hexachlorocychohexan, and methoxychlor), Erythrosine, FD&C Red No. 3, Nonylphenol, Polychlorinated biphenyls, Phenosulfothizine, Phthalates and Bis(2-ethylhexyl) phthalate (DEHP).[33]

---

[33] http://www.drjudyroth.com/

Liver detoxification is a central component of reestablishing the Progesterone to Estrogen ratio. Key factors for liver detoxification include:

(See Liver Toxicity section for additional recommendations)
- Start your day with ½ lemon squeezed in hot water.
- Consume ½ your body weight in filtered water each day.
- Consume liver cleansing foods on a daily basis such as beets, bitter greens, apples, lemons, flax seeds, garlic, cabbage and cruciferous veggies.
- Take liver clearing herbs such as Dandelion, Artichoke, Milk Thistle, Turmeric and Burdock root.
- Supplement with additional detoxifying fibers and herbs such as Apple pectin, flax seed, Triphala, glutamine, rice bran, beet fiber, oat fiber, psyllium, prune powder and sun fiber.
- Do a liver cleanse 2 times per year.

Herbal Medicine Indicated for Estrogen Dominance

Milk Thistle (*Silymarin marianus*)

Much research has been done on a special extract of milk thistle known as Silymarin which is a group of flavonoid compounds. These compounds protect the liver from damage and enhance the detoxification process. Silymarin prevents damage to the liver by acting as an antioxidant and is much more effective than vitamins E and C. Numerous studies have demonstrated its protective effect on the liver and it also works by preventing the depletion of glutathione. The higher the glutathione concentration, the greater the liver's capacity to detoxify harmful chemicals. Silymarin has been shown to increase the level of glutathione by up to 35%. In human studies, Silymarin has been shown to exhibit positive effects in treating liver diseases of various kinds including cirrhosis, chronic hepatitis, fatty infiltration of the liver and inflammation of the bile duct. Dosage: standardized extract 200 to 800 mg a day

Curcumin (*Curcuma longa*)

Several studies have illustrated curcumin's hepatoprotective effects. This has led researchers to suggest its use in protecting the liver from exogenous insults from environmental toxins including carbon tetrachloride and acetaminophen. Curcumin also has the capacity to increase bile flow and solubility, making it of potential benefit for someone with a tendency to form gallstones. The hepatoprotective effects of curcumin may stem from its potent antioxidant activity. In addition to its antioxidant effects, curcumin has been shown to enhance liver detoxification by increasing the activity of glutathione S-transferase which is an enzyme necessary to conjugate glutathione with a wide variety of toxins in order to facilitate their removal from the body. Dosage: 500mg-2000mg per day

Specific Nutrients for Estrogen Dominance

Diindolylmethane (DIM)

DIM is a powerful metabolizer of estrogen, assisting in removing excess estrogen and benefiting individuals with conditions associated with estrogen dominance. Supplementation with DIM can help promote proper estrogen levels in women through the pre and perimenopausal years as well as in men experiencing higher estrogen levels. These conditions include, but are not limited to, uterine fibroid tumors, fibrocystic breasts and glandular dysfunction. DIM can also benefit men by improving estrogen dominance related health issues such as hair loss, atherosclerosis, prostrate problems, lowered libido and impotency. DIM promotes testosterone action which improves mood, fights depression, boosts libido, improves cardiovascular health, improves memory and supports muscular development. DIM is a balancer of estrogen metabolism. It increases 2-hydroxyestrone (2-OHE) which is also known as the good or protective estrogen. Dosage: 70 mg to 400 mg per day

N-acetylcysteine (NAC)

N-acetylcysteine (NAC) is the precursor of both the amino acid L-cysteine and reduced glutathione (GSH). Animal and human studies of NAC have shown it to be a powerful antioxidant and a therapeutic agent for heavy metal toxicity and other diseases characterized by free radical, oxidative damage. As a source of sulfhydryl groups, NAC stimulates glutathione synthesis, enhances glutathione- S-transferase activity, promotes liver detoxification by inhibiting xenobiotic biotransformation and acts as a powerful nucleophile which is capable of scavenging free radicals. Historically, the most prevalent and well-accepted use of NAC has been as an antidote for acetaminophen (Tylenol) poisoning. The resultant liver toxicity is due to an acetaminophen metabolite that depletes the hepatocytes of glutathione and causes hepatocellular damage and possibly even death. NAC administered intravenously or orally within twenty-four hours of overdose is effective in preventing liver toxicity; however, improvement is most notable if treatment is initiated within eight to ten hours of acetaminophen overdose. NAC has also been effective for poisoning by carbon tetrachloride, acrylonitriles, halothane, paraquat, acetaldehyde, coumarin and interferon. In addition to its dramatic effects on liver poisoning, NAC is effective in promoting normal liver detoxification. Dosage: 350 mg to 2,000 mg a day

Calcium D-Glucarate

Calcium D-glucarate is a botanical extract found in grapefruit, apples, oranges, broccoli, spinach and Brussels sprouts. It is also made naturally in small quantities by the body. Scientists are discovering that it appears to protect against cancer and other diseases via a different mechanism than antioxidants such as vitamin C, carotenoids and folic acid. These vitamin antioxidants work by neutralizing toxic free radical damage in the body. However, there are other mechanisms by which the human body can detoxify itself such as conjugation and glucuronidation.

Conjugation and glucuronidation are detoxification processes that occur when toxins, carcinogens and used hormones are combined with and bound to water-soluble substances in the liver, thus making them easier to remove from the body. D-glucarate has been shown to support this vital process of removal by inhibiting an enzyme called beta-glucuronidase that can break bonds between toxins and used hormones allowing them to be re-circulated into the bloodstream rather than excreted.

D-glucarate may directly detoxify any environmental agents responsible for cancer formation. It has been postulated that D-glucarate exerts some of its effects by equilibrium conversion to D-glucarolactone which is a potent beta-glucuronidase inhibitor. This is one of the most important nutrients to enhance liver function. Dosage: 250 mg to 1,000 mg a day

Omega 3 Fatty Acids- Fish Oil

A diet low in fish oil has a decreased ratio of 2-(OH)-estrogen to 16-alpha-(OH)-estrogen and thereby, an increased cancer risk. Intake of fish oil also has been observed to inhibit the formation of human breast cancer cells in laboratory studies. Several theories have been proposed to explain the link between the high intake of fish oil and the low risk of cancer. Among the most important is the inhibition of eicosanoid production from arachodoinic acid and omega-6. Eicosanoids belong to a class of compounds that are derived from poly and saturated fatty acids including prostaglandins, hydroxyl, prostaglandins and leukotrienes. Prostaglandins are unsaturated fats and are a group of lipids made at sites of tissue damage or infection that are involved in dealing with injury and illness. They control processes such as inflammation, blood flow, formation of blood clots and the induction of labour. Prostaglandin E2 (PGE2) has been linked to the formation of several types of breast and prostate cancer. Tumor cells generally produce a large amount of AA derived from PGE2 and fish oil inhibits the oxidation of AA to PGE2. Eicosanoids derived from AA are also related to the modulation of estrogen metabolism. DHA has been shown to improve the response of breast tumors to cytotoxic agents. Dosage: 500 mg to 10,000 mg a day

Bioidentical Progesterone Cream

The USP progesterone used for hormone replacement comes from plant fats and oils, usually from a substance called diosgenin that is extracted from a very specific type of wild yam that grows in Mexico or from soybeans. In the laboratory, diosgenin is chemically synthesized into real human progesterone. The other human steroid hormones, including estrogen, testosterone, progesterone and the cortisones are also nearly always synthesized from diosgenin. Because progesterone is very fat-soluble, it is easily absorbed through the skin. Progesterone is absorbed into capillary blood from subcutaneous fat. Thus, absorption is best at skin sites where people blush such as the face, neck, chest, breasts, inner arms and palms of the hands. Dosage: For premenopausal women, the usual dose is 15 mg to 24 mg per day for fourteen days before expected menses, stopping approximately one day before menses. For postmenopausal women, the dose that generally works best is 15 mg per day for twenty-five days of the calendar month. (Bioidentical progesterone cream should contain 450 mg to 500 mg of progesterone per ounce and 900 mg to 1000 mg per two ounce container.)

Action Steps to Balance Estrogen Dominance

1. Get tested- Salivary testing will reveal the level of estrogen dominance in relation to progesterone.
2. Reduce and eliminate exposure to xenoestrogens.
3. Detox the liver- take a combination of Milk thistle, Dandelion root, Burdock root, Artichoke and Turmeric to detoxify excess estrogen.
4. Consume Cruciferous vegetables: broccoli, cauliflower, all cabbages, Brussels sprouts, kale, bok Choy, arugula, mustard greens and watercress.
5. Increase fiber intake to help expel excess estrogen- flax seeds, chia seeds, apple pectin, rice bran, psyllium, beet fiber, oat fiber and sun fiber.
6. Limit caffeine and alcohol consumption.
7. Go organic to limit the exposure of xenoestrogens through pesticides and hormone residue (most important are dairy, animal proteins and the Dirty Dozen-*see Organic Food section)*
8. Take estrogen detoxifiers: Diindolylmethane (DIM), Indole 3 carbinol (I-3-C), N-acetyl-cysteine (NAC), Calcium D-Glucarate, Green tea extract, Curcumin and Wasabia japonica.
9. Take Progesterone promoting herbs and nutrients: Chaste berry, Wild yam, Rehmannia root, Bupleurum root, Passion flower, Peony root and Coleus forskohlii.
10. Replace progesterone deficiency with Bio Identical Progesterone.
11. Regular exercise has been shown to increase Progesterone levels.

Food Allergies

Are Hidden Food Allergies Making You Fat?

Most people think of food allergies in terms of a severe reaction such as a child going into anaphylactic shock after exposure to peanuts. These types of reactions only account for 5% of people with food allergies. 95% of people with food allergies have "delayed onset" food allergies. These reactions cause symptoms anywhere from 30 minutes up to as much as 3 days after exposure to the offending foods. Many people are consuming allergenic foods several times per day. Each time they consume the food, the immune system goes into frenzy. As symptoms can be delayed up to 72 hours after eating the foods, the damage is often repeated over and over, meal after meal! Eventually inflammation seeps throughout the whole body, establishing an environment ripe for weight gain and chronic disease.

When the lining of the gut is in a constant state of inflammation, small holes open between the tightly woven cells that make up the walls of the gut. This leads to "leaky gut syndrome" which allows bacteria and partially digested food molecules to escape the protected digestive tract and enter the bloodstream. Once in the bloodstream, the immune system sets forth a full system attack as white blood cells surround the offending particle and systemic inflammation ensues. This inflammation is often not obvious but is like a smoldering fire created by the immune system as it tries to fend off a daily onslaught of food allergies.

Inflammation from any cause whether it is from a bacterial infection, a high sugar or high fat diet or from a food allergy will eventually cause insulin resistance which leads to increasingly high levels of circulating insulin. The higher the insulin level, the more fat that is stored around the mid-section.

In December 2007, a European study was published in an issue of *Diabetes* and it involved 2 groups of children-one group was normal weight and the other group was overweight. The objective of the study was to measure inflammation in 3 separate ways.

The 3 connecting factors for inflammation that were measured were deposits of plaque in the carotid artery, immune markers for delayed onset food allergies called Immunoglobulin G (IgG) and finally C-reactive protein (CRP), a general inflammatory marker was also monitored.

The results of the research was not what scientists had expected to see. The group of children that were overweight had very different test results than that of the normal weight group:

- CRP or general inflammation was 300% higher
- Signs of early atherosclerosis, an indicator of heart disease was present due to thicker carotid arteries
- Levels of IgG or the presence of food allergies was 250% higher

The outcome of the study was clear that in order to reduce inflammation and thus obesity, total elimination of food allergies must be part of the treatment plan.

Eating foods that you are allergic to can cause weight gain through inflammation. There is also a hormonal cascade of events that occur when the body is exposed to a food allergen.

When you eat a food to which you are allergic, your adrenal glands release the hormones cortisol and adrenalin to cope with the allergic reaction. Once these hormones are secreted, the liver is signaled to release and breakdown glycogen (stored carbohydrate) which results in elevated blood sugar levels. As the blood levels now have an increased level of blood sugar, the pancreas responds by increasing insulin in the bloodstream. Due to the high cortisol levels, your cells are directed to stop taking sugar up from the blood which causes temporary insulin resistance. Blood sugar levels remain high resulting in more insulin being released and the cycle continues.

Elevated insulin levels then activate the enzyme lipoprotein lipase which increases the production of fats. The consequence of the excess insulin is fat storage rather than fat burning for fuel. High insulin levels in the blood also inhibit the activity of the enzyme triglyceride lipase which breaks down stored fat for use as energy. Thus, if you have chronically high insulin due to continual exposure to food allergens, you cannot burn your own body fat. In addition, if your insulin level is high, the protein and carbohydrates you eat which are in excess of what you burn for fuel in the two hours after a meal are more likely to be converted and stored as fat.

Leptin, which is the body's master weight control hormone that signals the brain when the stomach is full is also affected by food allergies and the resulting inflammation. It is a well-established fact that overweight people usually have high levels of leptin but unfortunately the leptin does not always function properly. Just like insulin resistance can develop, so can leptin resistance. If an optimally healthy, normal-weight person overeats, their leptin level rises and this increases their metabolic rate and also decreases their appetite. If you have constant inflammation due to food allergies, this does not occur and leptin resistance ensues.

Common Symptoms of Hidden Food Allergies

Delayed onset or hidden food allergies are not always obvious but there are some very common symptoms that can occur:

- Weight gain
- Skin conditions

- Digestive symptoms
- IBS (Irritable Bowel Syndrome)
- Headaches
- Joint pain
- Asthma or other respiratory conditions
- Mood disorders
- ADD/ADHD

Two Ways to Identify Food Allergies

1. Blood testing called ELISA (enzyme-linked immunosorbent assay) can help to identify hidden food allergies. A simple blood test can uncover offending foods which should then be completely eliminated. IgG reactions also known as delayed onset reactions can take hours or days to develop. This makes it almost impossible to uncover which foods are causing the problem without testing. In an IgG reaction, the IgG antibodies attach themselves to the allergen and create an antibody-allergen complex. These complexes are normally removed by special cells called macrophages. However, if they are present in large numbers and the allergen is still being consumed, the macrophages can't keep up. The allergen-antibody complexes accumulate and are deposited in body tissues. Once in tissues, these complexes release inflammation causing chemicals that may contribute to disease.

2. An elimination diet can be very useful in determining allergenic foods. Eliminating the top inflammatory foods from the diet for a period of 3-6 weeks is difficult but the challenge is worth it. Foods to eliminate include dairy, gluten, soy, corn, eggs, citrus fruits, some nuts, nightshades (tomatoes, bell peppers, potato and eggplant) and other inflammatory foods *(see Elimination Diet Guidelines for details)*. After eliminating these foods for a set amount of time, each food is then re-introduced every 3 days to determine the sensitivities.

Elimination Diet Guidelines

FOODS TO INCLUDE	FOODS TO AVOID
FRUIT TO INCLUDE Strawberries, pineapple, apples, apricot, avocado, banana, blueberries, cherries, grapes, kiwi, mango, melons, nectarine, papaya, pear, peach, plums, prunes and raspberries Organically grown is always preferred.	**FRUIT TO AVOID** All citrus fruits (lemon, lime, orange, grapefruit, tangerine and clementine)
VEGETABLES TO INCLUDE Arugula, asparagus, artichokes, bean sprouts, bok choy, broccoli, Brussels sprouts, cauliflower, celery, cucumber, cabbage, endive, escarole, all types of greens and lettuce, green beans, jicama, mushrooms, okra, green peas, radishes, spinach, squash (summer and winter), sweet potatoes, taro, turnips, yams and zucchini All fresh, raw, steamed, grilled, sautéed, roasted or juiced Organically grown is always preferred.	**VEGETABLES TO AVOID** Corn Nightshades (Tomato, potato, eggplant, peppers, Goji berries and tomatillos)
GRAINS TO INCLUDE Rice (white, brown, sushi, wild), potatoes, oats (gluten-free), quinoa, millet, tapioca, amaranth and buckwheat	**GRAINS TO AVOID** Corn and all gluten-containing products including wheat, spelt, kamut, barley, rye and some oats
LEGUMES TO INCLUDE All legumes including peas and lentils (except soybeans)	**LEGUMES TO AVOID** soybeans, tofu, tempeh, soy milk, soy sauce and any product containing soy proteins
NUTS/SEEDS TO INCLUDE All nuts except peanuts – almonds, cashews, macadamia, walnuts, pumpkin seeds, brazil nuts and sunflower seeds—whole or as a nut butter	**NUTS/SEEDS TO AVOID** Peanuts, peanut butter and peanut oil

MEAT AND FISH TO INCLUDE All fresh or frozen wild fish (except shellfish) such as salmon, halibut, sole, mahi mahi, cod and snapper. Organic, hormone-free chicken, turkey, lamb and wild game (venison, buffalo, elk, etc.)	**MEAT AND FISH TO AVOID** Tuna, swordfish, shellfish, beef, pork, cold cuts, hot dogs, sausage and canned meats
DAIRY ALTERNATIVES Milk substitutes such as unsweetened rice, coconut and almond or other nut milk	**DAIRY AND EGGS TO AVOID** All dairy including milk, cheese, cottage cheese, cream, butter, yogurt, ice cream, non-dairy creamers, soymilk and eggs
FATS TO INCLUDE Cold pressed oils such as olive, flaxseed, sesame, walnut, hazelnut, pumpkin seed and coconut	**FATS TO AVOID** Margarine, butter, shortening, any processed or hydrogenated oils, peanut oil, mayonnaise and fried foods
BEVERAGES TO INCLUDE Filtered or distilled water, green tea, herbal tea, pure fruit juices, mineral water and roasted grain coffee substitutes	**BEVERAGES TO AVOID** Sodas and soft drinks (including sugar-free), alcoholic beverages, coffee, tea, or any other caffeinated beverages and sweetened fruit juice
SWEETENERS TO INCLUDE Brown rice syrup (gluten-free), chicory syrup, stevia, blackstrap molasses, fruit sweeteners such as Luo Han fruit, raw honey, pure maple syrup and yacon syrup	**SWEETENERS TO AVOID** White or brown sugar, high fructose corn syrup, Agave nectar, corn syrup, sucrose, dextrose, turbinado, nutritive corn sweetener and any artificial sweeteners, colors or flavors
HERBS/SPICES/CONDIMENTS TO INCLUDE Vinegars (except grain source), wasabi, mustard, horseradish, pesto (cheese-free) and all spices	**HERBS/SPICES/CONDIMENTS TO AVOID** High salt intake, chocolate, ketchup, relish, soy sauce, BBQ sauce, chutney, MSG, BHA, BHT, nitrates, nitrites and any other chemical additive or preservatives

The Challenge Phase of an Elimination Diet

After avoiding all problematic foods for a minimum of twenty one days, associated symptoms should be greatly diminished or eliminated. The purpose of the "challenge phase" of the elimination diet is to add back into the diet one new food every 3 days. During the first phase of food challenges, one new food is eaten one to three times during a 3 day period. This should be the only new food that is added back into the diet at this time. Over the next few days, a detailed account should be taken of any new or returning symptoms that occur.

If any symptoms develop, it is possible that there is an allergy or sensitivity to the recently reintroduced food. If no symptoms develop, it is likely that the reintroduced food is not a problem and the next new food can be reintroduced. In order to uncover hidden food allergies and food sensitivities, it is extremely helpful during the challenge phase to keep a diary of foods eaten and any emotional, mental or physical reactions.

Some of the specific symptoms that can occur during the challenge phase may include:
- insomnia
- mood swings
- energy fluctuations
- fatigue
- joint pain and/or inflammation
- skin breakouts or rashes
- headaches or migraines
- bowel changes
- intestinal cramping
- bloating or gas
- brain fog
- sinus or other respiratory issues

Gluten

Gluten is of particular importance when it comes to weight loss. There are actually four different ways that your body can negatively react to gluten exposure:

1. Celiac disease or Gluten intolerance
2. Non-Celiac gluten sensitivity
3. Delayed onset gluten allergy (elevated IgG gluten antibodies)
4. Immediate onset gluten allergy (elevated IgE gluten antibodies)

Gluten intolerance or Celiac disease has been found to be most common among people of Irish, Scottish, English, Scandinavian and Eastern European descent. A gluten intolerance is not an allergy but rather an autoimmune response which is becoming increasingly prevalent. The most significant symptoms are weight gain, mood disorders, fatigue, digestive issues and joint pain or inflammation.

The following test is a diagnostic tool designed by the Kalish Research Institute to help you to understand the symptoms and signs that are likely to go along with gluten intolerance.[34]

Test Interpretation Guide (combine both sections)

Number of "Yes" Responses   **Potential for Gluten Intolerance**

4 or less   →   Not likely

5-8   →   Suspected

9 or more   →   Very likely

Do any of the following apply to you?

	Yes	No
Weight gain		
Unexplained fatigue		
Difficulty relaxing, feel tense frequently		
Unexplained digestive problems		
Female hormone imbalances (PMS, Menopausal symptoms)		
Muscle, joint pain or stiffness of unknown cause		

---

[34] 2011 Dan Kalish www.kalishresearch.com

Migraine-like headaches		
Food allergies/sensitivities		
Difficulty digesting dairy products		
Tendency to over-consume alcohol		
Overly sensitive to physical and emotional pain, cry easily		
Craving for sweets, bread, carbohydrates		
Tendency to overeat bread, sweets, carbohydrates		
Abdominal pain or cramping		
Abdominal bloating or distention		
Intestinal gas		
"Love" specific foods		
Eat when upset, eat to relax		
Constipation or diarrhea of no none cause		
Unexplained skin problems/rashes		
Difficulty gaining weight		

Have you suffered from any of the following conditions?

	Yes	No
Allergies		
Depression		
Anorexia		
Bulimia		
Rosacea		
Diabetes		
Osteoporosis/Bone loss		
Iron deficiency/Anemia		
Chronic fatigue		
Irritable bowel syndrome		
Crohn's disease		
Ulcerative colitis		
Candida		
Hypoglycemia		
Lactose intolerance		
Alcoholism		

If you scored higher than 5 on the questionnaire, the recommendation is to completely eliminate gluten for a minimum of 3 months. If during this time your symptoms are eliminated, then the conclusion can be drawn that there is a reaction to gluten. Some people may want to confirm this sensitivity by reintroducing gluten back into the diet to see if the original symptoms return.

Gluten is the generic name for certain types of proteins contained in the common cereal grains wheat, barley, rye and their derivatives.

Gluten free grains:
- rice
- corn (maize)
- soy (should be fermented)
- potato
- tapioca
- beans
- garfava
- sorghum
- quinoa
- millet
- buckwheat
- arrowroot
- amaranth
- teff
- montina
- flax
- some oats
- nut flours

Grains containing gluten:
- wheat (einkorn, durum, faro, graham, kamut, semolina and spelt)
- rye
- barley
- triticale
- some oats

Foods/Products that may contain gluten:
- Beers, Ales and Lager
- Breading and Coating Mixes
- Brown Rice Syrup
- Communion Wafers
- Croutons
- Dressings
- Drugs and over-the Counter Medications
- Energy Bars
- Flour and Cereal Products
- Herbal Supplements
- Imitation Bacon
- Imitation Seafood
- Marinades
- Nutritional Supplements
- Pastas
- Processed Luncheon Meats
- Sauces and Gravies
- Self-Basing Poultry
- Soy Sauce or Soy Sauce Solids

- Soup Bases
- Thickeners (Roux)
- Vitamins and Mineral Supplements

The Damaging Effects of Gluten on the Body

In a case of gluten intolerance, Gliadin, the protein component of grains containing gluten cannot be properly digested. The enzyme transglutaminase is combined with gliadin when gluten is ingested and this forms an immune complex which is deposited on the intestinal lining. An immune reaction to the complex occurs because the body recognizes this as a foreign substance. Next, a series of toxins is released through the immune cells that flood the area in response to this unfamiliar immune complex. As a result the lining of the intestinal tract otherwise known as the "villi" is damaged from the consequential inflammation. This cascade of events causes a person to experience digestive symptoms such as gas, cramping, bloating, diarrhea, constipation as well as fatigue and malaise following a gluten containing meal.

As gluten is continually eaten, the immune system is further depleted. Secretory IgA (SIgA) immune cells which line the digestive tract for protection and defense against incoming attacks from bacteria, fungus and parasites is slowly broken down. The decreased SIgA leaves a person defenseless against these attacks. Malabsorption of nutrients also begins to occur as a result of the inflammation and resulting damage to the small intestine. Nutrient depletion then leads to fatigue and exhaustion.

As nutrients from food are no longer absorbed properly, the following issues may also arise such as:
- Osteoporosis due to calcium deficiency
- muscle cramping due to magnesium deficiency
- cardiovascular disease due to magnesium deficiency

- anxiety and restlessness due to mineral deficiencies
- insomnia due to mineral deficiencies
- weakness, fatigue and malaise due to B vitamin deficiencies
- peripheral neuropathy (numbness and tingling of extremities) due to B vitamin deficiencies
- anemia due to iron deficiency
- inflammation due to deficiency of healthy fats
- hormone imbalances due to deficiency of healthy fats
- weight gain due to resulting hormone imbalances
- diabetes due to insulin imbalance

In addition to deficiencies and the depletion of the SIgA cells that line the intestinal tract, the production of digestive enzymes becomes impaired. This impairment causes other food allergies to develop as the enzymes needed to break down foods properly are not in high enough levels. As this barrage of digestive impairment continues, the inability to breakdown protein can occur. Proteins in their simplest form are amino acids which are the building blocks for neurotransmitters, the brain messengers responsible for mood formation and stabilization. The main neurotransmitter is called Serotonin which is directly linked to mood disorders such as depression and sleep issues like insomnia.

Once a gluten free diet has been initiated, inflammation and damage to the lining of the intestinal tract can be completely reversed within three months to a year. The good news is that in time these issues can be conquered and total healing can take place.

Action Steps for Elimination of Food Allergies

1. Get tested- ELISA blood testing can help to determine delayed onset food allergies.
2. Do an elimination diet. For a minimum of 21 days, eliminate gluten, dairy, soy, eggs, shellfish, peanuts, citrus, nightshades, sugar, caffeine and alcohol.
3. If you suspect gluten is an issue, then eliminate it for a total of 3 months.
4. Take L-Glutamine to heal the intestinal lining.
5. Support the digestive system with probiotics.
6. Take digestive enzymes to assist with protein, fat and carbohydrate digestion.
7. Take a high quality multivitamin to replace deficiencies that result from food allergies.
8. Take Omega 3 fatty acids to restore depleted levels from fat malabsorption.
9. Supplement with extra magnesium if insomnia, restlessness or leg cramps are occurring.
10. Take additional calcium citrate with Vitamin D3 to protect against bone loss.

The Hidden Yeast Issue - Candida[35]

Candida albicans is a specific fungus or form of yeast found living in the intestinal tracts of most individuals. Candida can be an invasive problem that can drain energy stores, disrupt digestive function, deplete the immune system and cause the liver to be stressed as well as interrupt hormone balance and result in mood swings. People with Candida often suffer from the following common symptoms:

Common Symptoms of Candida

- **General**: chronic fatigue, sweet cravings, weight gain and skin conditions (acne, eczema and psoriasis)
- **Gastrointestinal system**: thrush, bloating, gas, intestinal cramps, rectal itching, alternating diarrhea and constipation
- **Genitourinary system**: vaginal yeast infections and frequent bladder infections
- **Hormonal system**: menstrual irregularities, PMS, menopause symptoms, fibroids and endometriosis
- **Nervous system**: depression, irritability, trouble concentrating and brain fog

---

[35] The Ultimate Candida Guide and Cookbook-Dr Cobi Slater, PhD, DNM, RHT, RNCP

- **Immune system**: allergies, chemical sensitivities, lowered resistance to infections and arthritis

The overuse of antibiotics as well as stressful conditions, damage to the intestinal tract, prescribed hormone treatments including birth control pills and hormone replacement therapy or immune system depression can all contribute to the overgrowth of Candida. Body processes are significantly disrupted as yeast cells and various toxic by-products of yeast metabolism easily enter general circulation.

Like most opportunistic infections, Candida overgrowth causes toxins to leak into the bloodstream or other tissues, allowing antigens (foreign substances) to invade bodily tissues. As an example a peanut is an antigen to a person who is allergic to peanuts. These antigens then trigger extensive allergic reactions which can lead to food, inhalant and environmental allergies. The major waste product of yeast cell activity is Acetaldehyde which is a poisonous toxin that promotes free radical activity in the body.

Yeasts cohabitate in a symbiotic relationship with over 400 healthy intestinal bacteria. These bacteria help produce short-chain fatty acids, vitamin K, biotin, vitamin B12, thiamin and riboflavin. The yeast in the intestinal tract is kept in balance by these bacteria. Problems arise when the yeast flourish beyond healthy levels. This occurs when these good bacteria die from antibiotics or are suppressed by prescription steroids.

Acetaldehyde is the major breakdown by-product of yeast cell activity. This is a toxin that is poisonous because it promotes free radical activity within the body. Acetaldehyde is also converted by the liver into ethanol which is in drinking alcohol. There are many people with Candida that experience a feeling of intoxication, brain fogginess and a hung- over feeling along with debilitating fatigue from the high amounts of ethanol in their system.

Once the yeast organism invades and attaches itself to the intestinal walls, nutrition is compromised and the body is depleted of vital nutrients. In addition, over 79 distinct antigens have been clearly identified because of the large number of mycotoxins (substances naturally produced by fungus) and antigens secreted by Candida. The immune system is greatly taxed as a result of this overgrowth of Candida.

Detailed Symptoms of Candida

Candidiasis can present a wide variety of symptoms and the exact combination and severity of Candida related symptoms are unique to each individual case. Candidiasis can manifest itself through many seemingly unrelated symptoms and therefore the diagnosis is very often missed.

General Symptoms	Inability to lose/gain weight Water retention Headaches/Migraines Heart palpitations Cravings for sweets and alcohol Chronic fatigue/Fibromyalgia Hypoglycemia Night sweats
Psychological	Inability to focus Poor memory/Brain Fog Insomnia Poor coordination Hyperactivity Mood swings Depression/Anxiety Dizziness
Digestive	Acid reflux Nausea Indigestion Mucus in stool Hemorrhoids Irritable bowel syndrome-Bloating/Gas/Cramping/Diarrhea/Constipation Excess weight centered around the abdomen Itching anus

Skin	Cysts Hives Skin conditions-Psoriasis, Eczema and Acne, Fungal infections of the nails, groin, inner ears, feet and skin Body odor Hair loss/Prematurely graying hair
Oral	Thrush (white coating on tongue) Swollen lower lip Metallic taste in mouth/Halitosis Canker sores Bleeding gums/Cracked tongue
Respiratory	Persistent cough/Asthma Mucus in throat/Sore throat Sinus congestion/Sinusitis Chronic post-nasal drip Flu-like symptoms
Eyes and Ears	Eye pain/Sensitivity to light Itchy eyes Blurred vision Dilated pupils Dark circles under eyes Ringing in the ears Ear infections
Genito-Urinary	Recurring yeast infections/Urinary Tract Infections Interstitial Cystitis (inflammation of the bladder) PMS (Pre Menstrual Syndrome) Endometriosis Low libido
Immune	Frequent colds and flu Environmental allergies Food allergies Sensitivity to fragrances, chemicals and smoke Autoimmune conditions
Musculoskeletal	Chronic body pain Joint pains Muscle aches and stiffness

Many experts agree that Candida is possibly the least understood and most widespread cause of chronic illness in modern day society. There are many people suffering from the symptoms of Candida without awareness that a single underlying cause could be to blame.

Testing Candida

Discovering if you have an overgrowth of Candida is crucial to overcoming any chronic condition. An excessive amount of Candida can destroy your health and quality of life in numerous ways. Many areas of the body can be affected such as the genital tract, digestive system, the heart, the brain, the liver, the joints and the eyes.

A Candida overgrowth has the ability to not only steal nutrients from the foods that you are consuming but also poison the tissues of the body with waste materials containing over 75 known toxins. The ravaging effects of this opportunistic yeast can manifest as numerous seemingly unrelated ailments.

As Candida flourishes, it plays into a larger problem called dysbiosis. Dysbiosis is the imbalance of the bacterial environment in the digestive tract. The army of "good" bacteria begins to dwindle because of poor dietary and lifestyle choices, stress, medications and a weakened immune system. The result is that the "bad" bacteria then flourishes.

Many conventional medical practitioners do not recognize Candida as a medical issue. This makes it one of the most overlooked and chronic health issues this generation has had to face. Diagnosing Candida is not an easy task for any health practitioner due to the lack of agreement over a definitive diagnostic test for intestinal yeast overgrowth. However, there are many tests available to determine if the possibility of Candida exists. Step one is to begin with the Candida questionnaire.

Candida Questionnaire

This candida test, a questionnaire created by Dr. William G. Crook when he published the first popularly read book on candida, "The Yeast Connection". This questionnaire has remained a standard in assessing candida related illness for many years.

A Candida self-test is one of the most useful and accurate methods of determining yeast-related health problems. It also serves as a tool for monitoring your health progress. Please answer all questions.

History	Point Score
1. Have you taken tetracycline or other antibiotics for acne for one month or longer?	25
2. Have you, at any time in your life, taken other broad-spectrum antibiotics for respiratory, urinary or other infections for two months or longer or in short courses four or more times in a one-year period?	20
3. Have you ever taken a broad-spectrum antibiotic?	6
4. Have you been pregnant. . .?	
One time?	3
Two or more times?	5
5. Have you, at any time in your life, been bothered by persistent prostatitis, vaginitis, or other problems affecting your reproductive organs?	25
6. Have you taken birth control pills. . .?	
For six months to two years?	8
For more than two years?	15
7. Have you taken prednisone or other cortisone-type drugs. . .?	
For two weeks or less?	6
For more than two weeks?	15
8. Does exposure to perfumes, insecticides, fabric shop odors, and other chemicals provoke. . .	
Mild symptoms?	5
Moderate to severe symptoms?	20

9. Are your symptoms worse on damp, muggy days or in mouldy places? — 20

10. Have you had athlete's foot, ringworm, "jock itch," or other chronic infections of the skin or nails?

    Mild to moderate? — 10

    Severe or persistent? — 20

11. Do you crave sugar? — 10

12. Do you crave breads? — 10

13. Do you crave alcoholic beverages? — 10

14. Does tobacco smoke really bother you? — 10

Total score of this section _____

Major symptoms

For each of your symptoms, enter the appropriate figure in the point score column.

Score Column

If a symptom is occasional or mild, score **3 points**.

If a symptom is frequent and/or moderately severe, score **6 points**.

If a symptom is severe and/or disabling score **9 points.**

Point Score

1. Fatigue or lethargy _____

2. Feeling of being "drained" _____

3. Poor memory _____

4. Feeling "spacey" or "unreal" _____

5. Depression _____

6. Numbness, burning or tingling _____

7. Muscle aches _____
8. Muscle weakness or paralysis _____
9. Pain and/or swelling in the joints _____
10. Abdominal pain _____
11. Constipation _____
12. Diarrhea _____
13. Bloating _____
14. Persistent vaginal itch _____
15. Persistent vaginal burning _____
16. Prostatitis _____
17. Impotence _____
18. Loss of sexual drive _____
19. Endometriosis _____
20. Cramps and/or other menstrual irregularities _____
21. Premenstrual tension _____
22. Spots in front of the eyes _____
23. Erratic vision _____

Total score of this section _____

Other symptoms

For each of your symptoms, enter the appropriate figure in the point score column.

Score column

If a symptom is occasional or mild, score **1 point**

If a symptom is frequent and/or moderately severe, score **2 points**

If a symptom is severe and/or disabling, score **3 points.**

	Point score
1. Drowsiness	_____
2. Irritability	_____
3. Lack of coordination	_____
4. Inability to concentrate	_____
5. Frequent mood swings	_____
6. Headache	_____
7. Dizziness/loss of balance	_____
8. Pressure above ears, feeling of head swelling/tingling	_____
9. Itching	_____
10. Other rashes	_____
11. Heartburn	_____
12. Indigestion	_____
13. Belching and intestinal gas	_____
14. Mucus in stools	_____
15. Hemorrhoids	_____
16. Dry mouth	_____

The Hidden Yeast Issue - Candida

17. Rash or blisters in mouth _____
18. Bad breath _____
19. Joint swelling or arthritis _____
20. Nasal congestion or discharge _____
21. Postnasal drip _____
22. Nasal itching _____
23. Sore or dry throat _____
24. Cough _____
25. Pain or tightness in chest _____
26. Wheezing or shortness of breath _____
27. Urinary urgency or frequency _____
28. Burning on urination _____
29. Failing vision _____
30. Burning or tearing of eyes _____
31. Recurrent infections or fluid in ears _____
32. Ear pain or deafness _____

Total score of this section _____

Total score of all sections _____

Interpretation

	Women	Men
Yeast-connected health problems are almost certainly present	≥180	≥140
Yeast-connected health problems are probably present	120-180	90-140

Yeast-connected health problems are possibly present	60-119	40-89
Yeast-connected health problems are less likely present	≤60	≤40

Lab Testing for Candida

Blood Test for Candida

An immunoglobulin test measures the level of certain immunoglobulins or antibodies, in the blood. Antibodies are proteins made by the immune system to fight antigens such as bacteria, viruses and toxins. IgA, IgG, and IgM are frequently measured simultaneously. Evaluated together, they can give health care practitioners important information about immune system functioning, especially relating to infection or autoimmune disease.

Blood analysis under powerful microscopes can be used to find Candida antibodies. When Candida takes on its fungal form, the immune system responds by producing special antibodies to fight off the infection. A large concentration of these antibodies in the blood is an indication of a Candidiasis overgrowth.

Candida Immune Complexes tests measure Candida specific IgG immune complexes. Immunoglobulin G (IgG), the most abundant type of antibody, is found in all body fluids and protects against bacterial and viral infections.

Stool Analysis for Candida

The stool is directly analyzed for levels of yeast, pathogenic bacteria and friendly bacteria. Stool analysis tests diagnose Candidiasis through a laboratory examination of a stool sample. If the stool contains abnormally large amounts of Candida then Candidiasis may be indicated.

A stool analysis can also look at other digestive markers for determining Candida levels such as:

- Levels of beneficial bacteria in the intestines
- pH levels in the stool

- Intestinal parasites, like worms and single-celled organisms such as blastocystis hominis and amoeba
- SIgA which is the state of your gut immune system (a low SIgA can indicate low immunity or gut inflammation)
- Leaky gut syndrome

Urine Tartaric Acid Test

This test detects tartaric acid which is a waste product of Candida yeast overgrowth. An elevated test means an overgrowth of Candida.

The Organic Acids Test (OAT)

The OAT provides an accurate evaluation of intestinal yeast and bacteria. Abnormally high levels of these microorganisms can be linked to behavior disorders, hyperactivity, movement disorders, fatigue and immune dysfunction. Many people with chronic illnesses and neurological disorders often excrete several abnormal organic acids. The cause of these high levels can include oral antibiotic use, high sugar diets, immune deficiencies and genetic factors.

Candida Urine Test

Secretory Immunoglobulin A (sIgA) test and intestinal permeability test can be taken to assess the permeability of the gut wall (leaky gut syndrome). This is associated with the development of food sensitivities and Candida infections in addition to a build-up of potentially damaging toxins.

Breath Hydrogen Test

Bacterial dysbiosis results from the same causes as a Candida overgrowth. This is a test for bacterial overgrowth, or intolerances to lactose, fructose or sucrose. The test measures the amount of hydrogen on a patient's breath within a specified amount of time after they have ingested a sugar solution. An elevated level of hydrogen indicates an overgrowth of bacteria in the small intestine. This test requires that you drink a solution of lactose, fructose, sucrose or glucose in water.

Complications of Candida

Leaky Gut Syndrome and Candida

Leaky Gut Syndrome is a weakening and inflammation of the intestinal wall. During Candida overgrowth the yeast cells attach themselves to the intestinal walls and actually penetrate through the membrane into the bloodstream.

As Candida cells and food particles enter the circulatory system, they provoke a strong immune response from the body and this triggers an inflammatory response of the intestinal wall. These Candida cells and food particles are foreign particles that do not belong in the blood. The immune system reacts quickly to destroy them by sending specialized immune cells known as macrophages. Next, the immune system creates antibodies ready for the next time it sees these same cells. The next time this particular food is consumed, an immune response is triggered. This hypersensitivity of the immune system is how allergies start.

Candida and Weight Gain

One of the symptoms of systemic Candida is weight gain or difficulty losing weight. It can cause the kind of stubborn fat deposits that are hard to shake off, no matter how little you eat or how much exercise you do. Candida cells are constantly reproducing and dying. The natural life cycle of this yeast results in toxins being released from dying Candida cells which are constantly being secreted into the bloodstream. The liver has to process these toxins and expel them from the body. If the liver becomes too burdened from too many toxins in the bloodstream, it has to accumulate these harmful chemicals to be processed later. This occurs because the liver stores them in fat cells primarily around the hips, belly and thighs. For many dieters, this is the root cause of abnormal fat deposits.

Sugar Cravings

Candida needs sugar to grow and reproduce. A typical symptom of a Candida infestation is increasingly severe sugar and carbohydrate cravings. The Candida yeast is consuming and burning large amounts of sugar and then sending blood sugar levels into hypoglycemia. This resulting low blood sugar triggers signals from your brain that you need to eat more and this results in overeating.

Once Candida overgrows in the large intestine where it is supposed to be in small amounts, it migrates upward into the small intestines where digestion and assimilation of all nutrients takes place. When the small intestine is overgrown with Candida, the digestion is inhibited because many of the beneficial bacteria in the small intestines that are needed for digestion as well as for your immune system are killed by the Candida.

Candida upsets the body's blood sugar as it seeks to be fueled by its primary food, sugar. Due to disrupted digestion by Candida, there is a lack of the minerals needed to escort sugar and insulin into the cells. This results in hypoglycemia as there are inadequate amounts of sugar entering the cells.

Due to the lack of minerals and low blood sugar tendencies which occur especially at night because the Candida has had a chance to burn through most of the sugar, the levels plunge even further. The brain then signals the adrenal gland to produce more adrenal hormones to keep the body functioning during the night. This can result in heightened cortisol and cause night sweats. The adrenal gland is now working overtime 24 hours per day and this leads to its eventual burn-out, resulting in adrenal fatigue. This depleted state of the adrenal glands further weakens the immune system leaving the body powerless and unable to fight Candida.

The Candida Elimination Protocol

Once a Candida diagnosis has been confirmed through the Candida questionnaire and/or one of the recommended lab tests, the protocol can begin for a minimum of three months. For the elimination of Candida to be successful, strict adherence to the plan is crucial. Candida is an opportunistic fungus and it will strike and flourish at any opportunity. The weakest strains are killed off initially and the stronger strains take more time to be eliminated. Therefore any variance while on the plan will only serve to strengthen the stronger strains of Candida which then render it much more difficult to treat.

Dietary Guidelines

Follow the dietary guidelines outlined in the "Do's and Don'ts" Food Lists.

Month 1- In addition to the dietary guidelines, eliminate all grains in all of their forms for a period of one month. After one month, only 1 cup of gluten free whole grains per day can be reintroduced. In some cases, complete elimination of grains is needed throughout the cleansing period. If after 1 month of the plan, there is not a complete elimination of symptoms, it is then recommended to remain grain free for the duration. No flour of any grain is allowed during the entire program. If grains are tolerable after the month elimination, then only whole grains are permitted (i.e. whole brown rice is allowable but brown rice flour is not).

Supplements

*all recommended supplements are available online at www.drcobi.com

During the Candida Protocol, the antifungals will be rotated each month to prevent any resistance from occurring. Candida has a tendency to become familiar with certain antifungals which causes them to stop working. Alternating the remedies each month will ensure that does not occur.

Choose one of the antifungals each month and take the full recommended dose. If any "die off" reactions occur during the first few weeks, decrease the dose by half and slowly work back up to the full dose. You can also utilize the remedies under the "die off" support list to help ease the detoxification symptoms.

Antifungals:

Caprylex (Douglas labs) (*Contains Caprylic acid*) - Take 1 to 3 tablets three times daily with food

Berbercap (Thorne) (*Contains Berberine HCl*) - Take 1 capsule two to three times daily with food

Anti-MFP (Douglas Labs)(*Contains: Grapefruit Seed Extract, Olive Leaf Extract, Berberine HCl, Burdock (root), Goldenseal (root), Black Walnut Hull Powder*) -Take 2 to 4 capsules daily with food

Grapefruit seed extract —Take 10 to 20 drops of liquid or 200 mg of powder or pills three times daily with food

Yeast Balance Complex (Integrative Therapeutics)(*Contains a comprehensive blend of Goldenseal, Pau d'arco, Milk thistle, Garlic, Barberry, Prebiotics, Probiotics and digestive enzymes*) -Take 1-2 caps three times daily with food

Formula SF722 (Thorne) (*Contains Undecylenic acid - from Castor beans*) -Take 5 gel caps three times daily with food

Candibactin AR (Metagenics) (*Contains Red Thyme oil, Oregano oil, Sage leaf, Lemon balm*) - Take 1 soft gel three times daily with food

Candibactin BR (Metagencis) (*Contains Coptis, Oregon grape, Berberine HCl, Chinese skullcap, Phellodendron bark, Gingerrhizome, Chinese licorice root, Chinese Rhubarb root and rhizome*)- Take 2 tablets two to three times daily with food

Oil of Oregano- 4 - 6 drops (about 50 mg. of 100% pure Oil of Oregano diluted with a carrier oil such as olive oil. A safe blend is 1 part oregano oil to 3 parts olive oil) - can also be used topically for yeast related rashes and infections

Other supportive antifungals which can be used in addition to the above mentioned remedies:
Coconut oil- Start with 1 teaspoon per day and work up to 5 teaspoons per day -can also be used topically for yeast related rashes and infections

Colloidal silver- Hold 1 teaspoon under the tongue for thirty seconds and swallow -can also be used topically for yeast related rashes and infections (do not use internally for longer than 30 days consecutively)

Bentonite Clay- It is generally advisable to start with 1 tablespoon of bentonite clay daily mixed with a small amount of water (pay attention to the results for a week and then gradually increase the dosage to no more than 4 tablespoons daily in divided doses)

Psyllium powder- 1/2 to 2 tsp. of psyllium powder into 8 oz. of water (drink an additional 8oz of water to prevent constipation from occurring)

Allium sativa (garlic) -An encapsulated supplement is sometimes necessary to deliver high enough concentrations to the intestines which will avoid irritating the stomach (also beneficial is to include one to three cloves of raw garlic in the diet daily)

Probiotics

Probiotics play a critical role in the elimination of Candida. The term 'probiotic' is derived from the Greek, meaning 'for life'. Probiotics are currently defined as 'live microorganisms which, when consumed in adequate amounts, confer a health benefit to the host. Common descriptions for probiotics include 'friendly', 'beneficial' or 'healthy' bacteria.

The beneficial bacteria contained in probiotics secrete small quantities of lactic acid and acetic acid. These help to maintain the correct levels of acidity in your stomach. This is important because the Candida yeast can switch to its pathogenic, fungal form in an alkaline environment, therefore restoring the stomach back to its normal acidity which will restrain the Candida overgrowth.

It is crucial to take Probiotics daily without food throughout the entire protocol. Probiotics are best taken before bed or first thing in the morning with a full glass of non-chlorinated water. Lactobacilli are probably the most important addition to the diet in combating a gastrointestinal yeast overgrowth. Both are taken by mouth or as rectal implants. Two strains are of significance Lactobacillus acidophilus (especially for upper GI) and Bifidobacterium bifidus (especially for the colon or large bowel).

Ultraflora Balance (Metagenics) (*Contains a dairy free patented probiotics blend of 15 billion of B.lactis Bi-07 and L. acidophilus NCFM which is the most well researched probiotic strain*) -Take 1 capsule one to two times per day on an empty stomach

Ultra Flora IB (Metagenics) (*Contains 60 billion strain-identified micro-organisms in a 50:50 ratio including B.lactis Bi-07 and L. acidophilus NCF*) - Take 1 capsule one to two times daily on an empty stomach

Sacro B (Saccharomyces boulardii) (Thorne) (*Contains a yeast species that can provide substantial support to the health of the gastrointestinal tract by supporting beneficial intestinal flora*) -Take 2 capsules two times daily on an empty stomach

Multi Probiotic 4000 (Douglas Labs) - *(Contains a combination of 15 billion organisms coming from 6 different strains and a pre-biotic blend)* - Take 1 to 2 capsules two time daily on an empty stomach

HMF Series Probiotics (Genestra):

HMF Candigen (*Contains two strains of Lactobacillus and garlic in a vaginal ovule form*) - Use 1 ovule per day at bedtime

HMF Candigen Cream-150 billion CFU per dose (*Contains two strains of Lactobacillus, Garlic and Rosa Damascena in a cream form*) - Apply a thin layer of cream to the external vaginal area two to three times daily

HMF Replete (*Contains a highly concentrated probiotic formula of two strains of Lactobaccillus acidophilus, Lactobacillus salivarius, Bifidobacterium bifidum and Bifidobacterium animalis lactis along with fructooligosaccharides*) -Take one sachet per day for 7 days on an empty stomach

HMF Replenish-100 billion CFU per dose (*Contains two strains of Lactobaccillus acidophilus, Lactobacillus salivarius, Bifidobacterium bifidum and Bifidobacterium animalis lactis along with fructooligosaccharides*) -Take 1 capsule daily on an empty stomach

HMF Intensive- 25 billion (*Contains two strains of Lactobaccillus acidophilus, Lactobacillus salivarius, Bifidobacterium bifidum and Bifidobacterium animalis lactis*) -Take 1 capsule per day on an empty stomach

Numbers 1, 2 and 3 consist of the basic fundamental treatment protocol. Numbers 4, 5, 6 and 7 include additional supportive nutrients that can be added to the fundamental protocol on an individual basis as needed.

	Month 1	Month 2	Month 3
1. Nutrition (additional detailed guidelines follow this chart)	No grains	0-1 cup Gluten free grains in their whole form only (NO GRAIN FLOURS)	0-1 cup Gluten free grains in their whole form only (NO GRAIN FLOURS)
2. Probiotics	Choose one: (to be taken throughout) - HMF Replete (first 7 days only) - Ultra Flora Balance - Sacro B - Multi Probiotic 4000 - HMF Replenish - HMF Intensive	Choose one: (to be taken throughout) - Ultra Flora Balance - Sacro B - Multi Probiotic 4000 - HMF Replenish - HMF Intensive	Choose one: (to be taken throughout) - Ultra Flora Balance - Sacro B - Multi Probiotic 4000 - HMF Replenish - HMF Intensive
3. Anti Fungals	Choose one and rotate each month: - Caprylex - Berbercap - Anti-MFP - Grapefruit Seed Extract - Yeast Balance Complex - Formula SF 722 - Candi Bactin AR - Candi Bactin BR - Oil of Oregano	Choose one and rotate each month: - Caprylex - Berbercap - Anti-MFP - Grapefruit Seed Extract - Yeast Balance Complex - Formula SF 722 - Candi Bactin AR - Candi Bactin BR - Oil of Oregano	Choose one and rotate each month: - Caprylex - Berbercap - Anti-MFP - Grapefruit Seed Extract - Yeast Balance Complex - Formula SF 722 - Candi Bactin AR - Candi Bactin BR - Oil of Oregano
4. Other Supportive Yeast Killers	Choose two: - Coconut oil - Colloidal Silver - Bentonite Clay - Psyllium Powder - Garlic	Choose two: - Coconut oil - Colloidal Silver - Bentonite Clay - Psyllium Powder - Garlic	Choose two: - Coconut oil - Colloidal Silver - Bentonite Clay - Psyllium Powder - Garlic
5. Die Off Support	As needed, usually only in Month 1: - Psyllium - Bentonite Clay - Medibulk - Metafiber - Molybdenum - HTC		

6. Immune Support	Choose two and take throughout or more: - Vitamin D3 - Vitamin A - Zinc - Selenium - Omega 3	Choose two and take throughout or more: - Vitamin D3 - Vitamin A - Zinc - Selenium - Omega 3	Choose two and take throughout or more: - Vitamin D3 - Vitamin A - Zinc - Selenium - Omega 3
7. Liver Support	Choose one: - LVDTX - LCH - SAT - TAPS - Cyste Plus - Calcium D Glucarate	Choose one: - LVDTX - LCH - SAT - TAPS - Cyste Plus - Calcium D Glucarate	Choose one: - LVDTX - LCH - SAT - TAPS - Cyste Plus - Calcium D Glucarate
8. Digestive Support	Choose one and take throughout: - BPP - Bio Gest - Dipan 9 - Ultrazyme - Plantizyme	Choose one and take throughout: - BPP - Bio Gest - Dipan 9 - Ultrazyme - Plantizyme	Choose one and take throughout: - BPP - Bio Gest - Dipan 9 - Ultrazyme - Plantizyme

Candida Control Diet Guidelines- Minimum 3 Months

Category	To Include	To Exclude
Fruits	2 servings of domestic fruit only (berries, peaches, plums, apples, apricots, pears)	All dried fruits, juices and tropical fruits
Eggs, dairy, & dairy replacement	Eggs; plain unsweetened yogurt (cow, sheep, or goat) unsweetened coconut/almond milk, unaged goat cheese	Cheese, milk, sour cream, sweetened yogurt, butter
Grains	None (month 1) or Gluten free (brown rice, quinoa, tapioca, millet, buckwheat, amaranth, teff, gluten free whole oats) **whole grains only. Only flours allowed**- coconut flour and almond meal	All refined or whole grains flours, breads, baked goods, products made with flour (except coconut/almond)
Flesh foods	Fish (fresh or canned) & other seafood, chicken, turkey, lean beef, lamb, (preferably organically-raised meats)	Cold cuts and all processed meats, pork
Meat Replacements	Non- GMO tofu, tempeh	None
Beans	In small amounts, any dried beans, split peas, and legumes (not more than 1 cup (cooked)/day)	None
Nuts & seeds	Walnuts, hazelnuts, filberts pecans, almonds, cashews, flax seeds, pumpkin seeds, sunflower seeds, poppy seeds sesame seeds – whole or as nut butters	Peanuts and pistachios
Vegetables	Non-starchy vegetables – raw, steamed, sautéed, juiced or baked	Mushrooms and starchy vegetables: potatoes, corn, yams, sweet potatoes, parsnips, cooked beets
Fats and oils	Coconut oil, avocado, olives, cold pressed oils: olive, flax seed, sesame, pumpkin, almond, walnut	Margarine, shortening, processed oils, prepared salad dressings, spreads, sauces, mayonnaise

Acidic & fermented foods	Lemon and lime juices and vitamin C crystals as replacements for vinegar.	All vinegars and preserved foods: sauerkraut, pickles, other products preserved in brine or vinegar
Sweeteners	Stevia (herbal sweetener), Xylitol	All: sugar, white/brown sugars, honey, maple syrup, corn syrup, high fructose corn syrup, molasses, brown rice syrup, fruit sweeteners
Beverages	Filtered, spring, or distilled water (drink 8 cups per day), herbal tea, green tea	Soda pop, juice, alcohol, black tea, coffee, non-dairy creamers

Action Steps to Eliminate Candida

1. Take the Candida Questionnaire.
2. Get tested to determine the level of Candida that is present.
3. For a minimum of 90 days, follow the Candida dietary guidelines.
4. Restore beneficial bacteria levels by supporting the body with high quality probiotics.
5. Detoxify yeast with antifungals-rotate antifungals each month *(choose from the outlined list of antifungals)*.
6. Support the body if needed during the "die off" phase.
7. Support the immune system with Vitamin D3, Zinc, Selenium, Vitamin A and Omega 3's.
8. Assist in liver detoxification by taking Milk thistle, Dandelion root, Burdock root, Artichoke, Calcium D-glucarate and N-acetyl cysteine (NAC).
9. Support the digestive system with digestive enzymes to aid in the breakdown of protein, fats and carbohydrates.
10. Take additional fiber to maintain optimal elimination- ground flax seed, psyllium, chia seeds, apple pectin and sun fiber.

The Sleep Connection

Sleep is one of the most important foundational aspects to achieving and maintaining a healthy weight. Sleep is like nutrition for the brain. Most people need between 7 and 9 hours each night.

In 2006 a study that followed more than 68,000 women for 16 years looked at the "Association between Reduced Sleep and Weight Gain in Women". It found that those who slept five hours or less a night were more likely to gain more weight than those who got seven hours of sleep a night. Insufficient sleep dulls brain activity, specifically in the frontal lobe which is responsible for impulse control and decision making. This can most certainly lead to poor decisions due to a lack of mental clarity when it comes to food choices. In addition to the dampening of the frontal lobe, the brain's reward center is stimulated when there is a lack of sleep. Stimulation of this area causes a person to look for something to make them feel good and this is often sugar and carbohydrate laden foods that feel comforting.

A study in the American Journal of Clinical Nutrition found that when people were starved of sleep, late-night snacking increased and they were more likely to choose high-carb snacks. In fact a review of 18 studies revealed that a lack of sleep led to increased cravings for high carbohydrate foods.

There are 2 very important hormones that control our appetite center and a lack of sleep can cause an imbalance in these hormones leading to weight gain and/or weight resistance. Sleep deprivation increases a hormone called ghrelin which triggers appetite and decreases one called leptin which signals that you are full.

Leptin and Ghrelin are secreted in the peripheral areas of the body but their effects are directly on the brain.

Leptin's effect is to decreases hunger and it is secreted primarily in fat cells as well as the stomach, heart, placenta and skeletal muscle. The amount of Leptin in the body strongly correlates with the amount of fat as it is produced by adipose tissue (fat tissue). Leptin communicates with the hypothalamus which is located in the brain that we are full and then that message will be sent down to the stomach. Once the message has been received, we stop eating. There is also some research to show that Leptin may also increase the metabolism. [36]

It would therefore seem that the more fat mass a person has, then more corresponding Leptin would be produced. Seemingly, this would be a benefit as the person would have a decreased appetite and a higher metabolic rate resulting in weight loss. However, most often something called Leptin Resistance develops.[37] This resistance causes the brain to ignore the increasing amounts of Leptin trying to signal the hypothalamus and the result is communication breakdown. Therefore the metabolism is slowed, the hunger is stimulated and weight gain continues.

Ghrelin, discovered 7 years after Leptin, increases hunger and is secreted primarily in the lining of the stomach. The function of Ghrelin is shorter acting than its counterpart Leptin as it is only high right before eating to stimulate hunger and is then decreased after a meal. Ghrelin also acts on the hypothalamus which then communicates that you are hungry.

The following picture depicts the actions of leptin and ghrelin:[38]

---

[36] Klok MD, Jakobsdottir S, Drent ML. The role of leptin and ghrelin in the regulation of food intake and body weight in humans: a review. Obes Rev. 2007 Jan;8(1):21-34. Review.

[37] Woods SC. The control of food intake: behavioral versus molecular perspectives. Cell Metab. 2009 Jun;9(6):489-98. Review.

[38] http://www.precisionnutrition.com/leptin-ghrelin-weight-loss

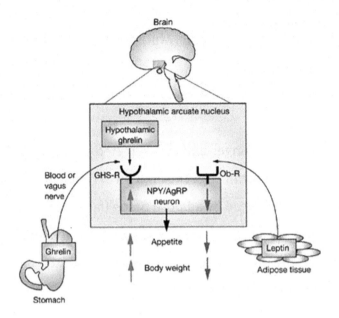

Signs of Sleep Disturbances

Difficulty sleeping can be a short term situation or can turn into a chronic problem. **The following list describes issues related to chronic sleep disturbances:**

- Difficulty falling asleep
- Difficulty waking up in the morning
- Daytime drowsiness
- Micro sleeps or "nodding off"
- Zoning out in a conversation or task
- Altered memory or judgment
- Difficulty concentrating
- Difficulty making simple decisions
- Clumsy and/or slower reaction times
- Feeling emotional for no apparent reason

- Snoring (sleep apnea)
- Routinely falling asleep within 5 minutes of lying down
- Waking up frequently during the night with difficulty returning to sleep

Testing for Chronic Sleep Issues

There are numerous underlying causes of sleep disturbances. ZRT Laboratory in Oregon, USA has been able to identify several patterns of hormonal imbalances that can cause sleep abnormalities. ZRT's Sleep Profile is specifically testing for the effects of stress on the sleep cycle. The stress hormone Cortisol which is released in our bodies during times of elevated stress can interfere with our capacity to sleep. Also featured in this profile is Melatonin, the well-known sleep hormone. The production of Melatonin begins to decline with age and can also become impaired due to elevated cortisol levels. For optimum health, cortisol and melatonin need to be in perfect balance with each other. The symphony of these two hormones plays out in a back and forth balancing rhythm. Top of FormWhen cortisol is high, melatonin should be low and when melatonin is high, cortisol should be low.

Included in the ZRT Sleep Profile:
- 4 specifically timed Cortisol readings (C x 4)
- 4 specifically timed Melatonin readings (MT6s x 4)

If two or more of these symptoms persist, testing can identify whether it's a hormone imbalance:
- can't get to sleep or stay asleep
- frequent or early waking
- morning or evening fatigue
- feeling "tired but wired"
- high stress

- irritability / impaired performance
- hunger / sugar cravings
- weight gain

Simple testing can reveal whether hormones are the hidden barrier to your restful sleep.

Tips for Sleeping Well

Below are some tips to help you get the sleep you need. It is also important to remember that getting too much sleep (over 9 hours) can be just as unhealthy.

- Consistently maintain regular bedtime and wake-up hours as much as possible.
- Aim for 7-9 hours of sleep per night.
- Get to bed no later than 11pm- go to bed 15 minutes earlier each week until you reach no later than 11pm.
- Avoid caffeine consumption (tea, cola, coffee, chocolate) within 4 to 8 hours of bedtime.
- Exercise regularly.
- Avoid daytime naps.
- Avoid eating a meal 3 hours before bedtime (a light snack can help avoid hunger pangs and aid sleep).
- Avoid alcohol as the body metabolizes alcohol while we sleep- even just one ounce within 2 hours of bedtime will disrupt sleep.
- Avoid stressful or noisy distractions while trying to sleep (noisy clocks, bright lights, uncomfortable clothes or bedding).
- Create a relaxing bedtime routine.
- Take a relaxing bath with lavender and chamomile aromatherapy added to the bath water.

- Turn the lights down low throughout the house or light candles. Turn off the screens as the electromagnetic rays from computer screens, TVs etc. are very stimulating.
- Make sure your room is as dark as possible-turn alarm clocks away from your head- use blackout curtains if light is entering from windows.
- Take the heat out- maintaining an average of 21°C (70°F) in the bedroom has been shown to be the best temperature for the production of the sleep inducing hormone melatonin.
- Remove clutter- keep your bedroom as neat and clutter free as possible.
- If you get up to go to the bathroom during the night, keep the lights off- any light that enters the iris of the eye can shut down melatonin production.
- Keep a journal- if endless mind chatter is keeping you up, then write down your thoughts or to do lists in a bedside journal to allow your mind to calm down.
- Sleeping with pets or children can be very disruptive to sleep- have them sleep in their own beds.
- Use the bed for sex and sleep only (no TV, laptop computer etc.).

Some very beneficial natural supplements and herbs for restoring sleep balance are:

GABA is a neurotransmitter or brain chemical that has a calming effect. Supplementing with GABA is indicated for people who suffer with anxiety, stress, muscle tension or pain. The recommended dose is 500mg-1000mg at bedtime. GABA can also be taken throughout the day for daytime anxiety which will disrupt nighttime sleep- 200-500mg up to 4 times per day.

Melatonin is produced by the pineal gland in the brain and is the main sleep inducing hormone. Supplementing with melatonin will only work if there is a deficiency present. Taking too much melatonin can result in vivid dreams or nightmares. Melatonin is extremely beneficial in the aging population as the melatonin production naturally slows with age. It is also effective in shift workers. Dosages range from 0.5mg up to 10mg before bed. Testing is available to reveal Melatonin deficiencies *(check the Appendix for lab recommendations)*.

5-HTP is used in the creation of Serotonin and is a derivative of Tryptophan. 5-HTP is very useful in the case of insomnia related to depression or anxiety. A natural side effect is that 5-HTP reduces appetite and is effective in reducing emotional eating. Dosing can be taken throughout the day with food or before bed. Recommended doses range from 100mg up to 400mg per day.

Relora is a combination of the herbs *Magnolia officinalis* and *Phellodendrum amurense.* Relora is very beneficial in the reduction of stress and anxiety as it balances the stress hormones cortisol and DHEA. It is helpful in the case of frequent nighttime awakenings due to stress and menopausal symptoms such as night sweats. Relora has been shown to also help to reduce belly fat as it lowers cortisol levels. Recommended dosages range from 250mg- 750mg taken in divided doses during the day and before bed.

Herbal combinations of **Valerian, Passion Flower, Hops** and **Lemon balm** have gentle yet powerful effects on sleep. They assist in the transition into a restful sleep but do not induce morning grogginess. Herbs such as these have been shown to be useful in situations of stress, anxiety and muscle tension. They have a calming effect on the nervous system making them useful in situations of over stimulation. Dosages vary depending on formulation *(see Appendix for recommended products)*

Phosphatidylserine is a stress hormone stabilizer and a cortisol lowering agent that helps to reduce stress and relieve occasional sleeplessness. This safe, natural and non-habit forming phospholipid increases the ability to fall asleep, stay asleep and will not cause morning grogginess while providing stress reduction all day.

Casein Hydrolysate (LactiumPure)

LactiumPure is a patented, bioactive decapeptide which research suggests promotes a healthy response to stress. In clinical studies, this unique ingredient was shown to boost the body's ability to manage stress and improve stress response measures including physical and emotional reactions. Research suggests that LactiumPure may influence the metabolism of cortisol which is the stress hormone as well as having a positive effect on the calming neurotransmitter GABA. Recommended dosages range from 75mg-300mg per day.

Action Steps for Restoring Sleep

1. Get tested - if sleep problems persist, testing can uncover the root causes.
2. Establish a relaxing bedtime routine.
3. Avoid caffeine and alcohol.
4. Avoid day time naps.
5. Create an optimal sleep environment.
6. Exercise regularly but not within 3 hours of bedtime.
7. Take Melatonin (start with 1mg and move up to a maximum of 5mg before bed).
8. Take 200-500mg of GABA, 300mg of Relora or 100-300mg of 5-HTP before bedtime if anxiety and stress are preventing sleep.
9. Take Phosphatidylserine (PS) if your nighttime cortisol levels are elevated.
10. Take a combination of Valerian, Passion flower, Hops and Lemon balm for a gentle, yet powerful sleep aid.

The Detrimental Effects of Sugar

The average North American consumes more than 100 pounds of sugar a year! From that number it sounds like everyone's polishing off a bag of cookies every day but the truth is, we are consuming many foods with a high sugar content that may not always be obvious. Many foods are deceiving and often we have no idea that they are loaded with that much sugar. It is time to get the skinny on sugar packed foods and learn how to dramatically decrease your consumption of white death (aka sugar)!

Many people have a very difficult time processing sugar in the body. Once a person has been exposed to chronically high levels of sugar over a period of time, symptoms of blood sugar instability can begin to manifest in the body.

Blood Sugar Instability Questionnaire

The following questionnaire designed by the Kalish Institute will determine if you have issues with sugar instability:[39]

Do any of the following apply to you?	Yes	No
Family history of diabetes, hypoglycemia or alcoholism		

---

[39] Dr Dan Kalish www.kalishresearch.com

Calmer after meals		
Frequent thirst		
Night sweats		
Crave salty foods		
Dark circles under eyes or eyes sensitive to bright light		
More awake at night		
Food cravings		
Headaches		
Irritability		
Mood swings		
Easily fatigued		
Anxiety		
Difficulty sleeping		
Mental sluggishness		
Eat when nervous		
Excessive appetite for carbohydrates or sweets		
Hungry between meals		
Irritable before meals		
"Shaky" if hungry		
Light headed if meals are skipped		
Low energy in the afternoon		
Afternoon headaches		
Crave sweets or coffee in the afternoon		

If you are experiencing more than 5 of these symptoms on a regular basis, this indicates that you are having issues with blood sugar instability. It is highly recommended that all sources of refined sugar be eliminated from the diet.

The Damaging Effects of Sugar on Your Health

In the book, "Lick the Sugar Habit" by Nancy Appleton, the detrimental effects of sugar on the body are explored in detail. The following is a detailed list of the many ways that sugar can damage the entire body.

Sugar has the following effects on the body:

- Suppress the immune system
- Upset the body's mineral balance
- Can cause anxiety
- Difficulty concentrating
- Decreases insulin sensitivity
- Decreases glucose tolerance
- Can increase cholesterol
- Can increase systolic blood pressure
- Interferes with protein absorption
- Can deplete chromium levels
- Elevate glucose and insulin responses in oral contraceptive users
- Can cause periodontal disease
- Can cause crankiness and hyperactivity in children
- Contributes to Osteoporosis
- Can cause a rise in Triglycerides
- Decreases growth hormone
- Can cause kidney damage
- Can reduce helpful, high density lipoproteins (HDL)
- Can increase harmful, low density lipoproteins (LDL)
- Can cause food allergies

Can cause copper deficiency

Can lead to diabetes

Can cause eczema

Can impair DNA structure

Can cause cataracts

Can cause arteriosclerosis

Can increase fasting glucose

Can weaken eyesight

Can cause varicose veins

Can cause hypoglycemia

Can cause stomach acidity

Can raise adrenal levels

Speeds the aging process

Stresses the pancreas

Can lead to alcoholism

Promotes tooth decay

Causes weight gain

Can cause tendon brittleness

Can cause toxemia during pregnancy

Interferes with the absorption of calcium and magnesium

Can lead to cardiovascular disease

May lead to cancer (breast, ovarian, prostate, colon or rectal)

Can cause emphysema

Can be a risk factor in gall bladder cancer

Can cause free radical damage

May lower the enzymes ability to function

Can cause loss of tissue, elasticity and function

Raises serotonin which can narrow blood vessels

Can cause liver damage/ fatty liver

Can indirectly cause hemorrhoids

Can cause blood platelet adhesiveness leading to blood clots

Can exacerbate the symptoms of multiple sclerosis

Can cause constipation

Can cause myopia (near sightedness)

Can compromise the lining of the capillaries

Can increase the risk of developing crohn's and colitis

Can cause headaches and migraines	May Inflame ulcers of the stomach
Can causes arthritis	Can cause depression
Can cause asthma	Can cause Candida
Increases colon bacterial formation	Can lead to the formation of kidney and gallstones
Can causes hormonal imbalance	Can cause appendicitis

The following are ten simple steps to reduce sugar consumption:

1. **Stop adding it to foods.** This is the easiest way to immediately reduce the amount of sugar you are consuming. The biggest targets are cereal, coffee and tea.
2. **Don't be fooled by "healthy sugar" disguises.** Brown sugar, turbinado sugar or raw sugar . . . it's all pretty much the same thing as far as your body is concerned. Reach for healthier proven alternatives such as green leaf stevia, xylitol, date sugar, raw honey or brown rice syrup.
3. **Beware of artificial sweeteners.** Unfortunately, they can increase cravings for sugar and carbohydrates. In addition, they can also deplete the body's stores of chromium which is a nutrient crucial for blood-sugar metabolism. Aspartame is one of most deadly toxins that we can consume. It is considered to be a "cumulative" toxin which means that even if you only have it a few times a week, it will build up in your body. It has the ability to cross the blood brain barrier and breaks down into formaldehyde!
4. **Don't be fooled by "fat-free" snacks.** Fat-free does not mean calorie-free. In addition, most of these snacks are loaded with sugar which turns into fat in your body.
5. **Think twice before getting your morning "fix".** The combination of supersizing and add-ins has made coffee house drinks a sugar and calorie magnet. Even buzzwords like "green tea" and "strawberry" shouldn't make you think of a healthy drink. A large size, typically 20 ounces or more, of many blended "frappe" type drinks can contain nearly 20 teaspoons of sugar. When it comes to these super-sweet drinks, always downsize to a small and skip

the sweetened whipped cream. You don't have to give up your morning latte, just make it a small skinny one!

6. **Reduce or eliminate processed carbohydrates.** Processed carbs such as breads, bagels, most pastas and snacks are quickly converted to sugar in the body. That sugar gets stored as triglycerides which is a fancy way of saying fat!

7. **Become a label reader.** To reduce sugar, you have to first know where it is lurking, so read labels and if any form of sugar is in the first few ingredients, then don't buy it! Better yet, don't buy anything in a package!

8. **Do the math**. 4 grams of sugar is equal to 1 teaspoon of sugar. That means that a small serving of fruit flavored yogurt contains 8-10 teaspoons of sugar and the newly popular Arizona Green Tea contains a staggering 50 grams of sugar which translates into 12.5 teaspoons of sugar!

9. **Skip the sauce!** Teriyaki and BBQ sauces are tangy with a touch of sweetness to taste but the sugar content packs a wallop. While switching to teriyaki flavoring instead of a fried chicken dish (from entrees to sandwiches to veggies) sounds healthy, one serving of teriyaki chicken packs a whopping 10 to 12 teaspoons of sugar per serving. Control the amount of sauce by asking for it on the side or skip it altogether. Steer clear of bottled teriyaki sauces for use at home and flavor your chicken or other meats with natural herbs and spices.

10. **Eliminate fruit juice.** It's a pure sugar hit with none of the fiber and less of the nutrients that are found in the fruit itself. While 100 percent juice does provide some vitamins and minerals, it's always better to eat your fruit of choice and not drink it. If you must drink fruit juice, then try to limit it to no more than 2 ounces per serving which is the approximate amount found in a piece of fruit.

Beware of Sneaky Sugars

The following table outlines the complete spectrum of sugars:

Avoid these Sneaky Sugars	Consume these Natural Sugars in Moderation
Artificial Sweeteners: • Aspartame (Equal, NutraSweet) • Saccharine (Sweet'N Low) • Sucralose (Splenda) • Acesulfame K/Acesulfame Potassium (Sweet One, Sunett) • White/Bleached Stevia (Truvia, Sun Crystals) **Naturally Derived Sweeteners:** • Agave nectar • Barley Malt • Corn Syrup • Demerara sugar • Dextrose • Fructose • Glucose • Golden sugar • Grape sugar • High fructose corn syrup • Maltitol • Malt syrup • Maltodextrin • Maltose • Mannitol • Sorbitol • Sorghum syrup • Sucrose • Yellow sugar	**Safest Natural Sweeteners:** • Green leaf Stevia • Stevia Extract • Coconut nectar • Coconut palm sugar • Date sugar • Date syrup • Raw honey • Pure Maple Syrup • Black strap molasses **Natural Sweeteners to be consumed in limited quantities:** • Cane juice • Cane juice crystals • Dates • Fruit juice • Raw sugar • Turbinado • Xylitol

Insulin Resistance

The pre-diabetic disposition in people today has become staggeringly high. According to Dr Prab R. Tumpati, MD, a practicing obesity medicine physician and founder of W8MD Medical Weight Loss Centers of America, the current diet which is very high in refined carbohydrates contributes significantly to this phenomenon of insulin resistance. [40]

Insulin is a hormone that is produced in the pancreas. The action of insulin is to control glucose or the blood sugar levels in the body. Glucose is our main source of fuel which allows our body to produce energy. Insulin helps to maintain balanced levels of blood sugar and is secreted in varying amounts depending on what we eat. The higher the carbohydrate or sugar content of the food, the greater the level of circulating insulin.

Glucose, or sugar, is absorbed by the cells of the body and is utilized for energy. Insulin signals the cells to allow the glucose into the cells. This is much like a lock and key receptor with insulin working as the key to open the lock which allows the sugar into the cells. Cells become desensitized when too much glucose is in the bloodstream. Blood sugar levels become increasingly high as the body continues to release more corresponding insulin.

High levels of insulin continues to knock on the door like the boy who cried wolf and eventually the cells quit responding to the insulin signal and this results in insulin resistance. The cells are so overwhelmed by the high levels of insulin that they reduce the amount of insulin receptors

---

[40] http://www.slideshare.net/philadelphiamedicalweightloss/insulin-resistancec

they have in order to protect themselves. Damage to the cardiovascular system occurs when high levels of insulin that have been forbidden by the cells are floating in the bloodstream.

Diabetes is the most common result of the effects of insulin resistance because the body is no longer able to manage the blood glucose levels.

As the cell walls are desensitized to insulin, the conversion of glucose into energy has now become compromised. Blood sugar levels are elevated as excess glucose permeates the bloodstream and is then sent to the liver. The liver then coverts the excess sugar to fat which is then deposited throughout the body via the bloodstream and this results in weight gain as well as obesity.

It is a well-established fact that a diet high in simple carbohydrates found in refined and processed foods has a negative result on blood sugar levels. The glucose in this type of food causes a very quick rise in blood sugar as well as a surge of insulin. The rate at which we burn energy, otherwise known as metabolism, has a first line effect on how glucose functions. A diet that is rich in vegetables, complex carbohydrates, low glycemic fruits and high fiber foods helps to support the metabolic processes in the body by slowly releasing small amounts of sugar into the blood.

Signs of insulin resistance

The number of people with insulin resistance is at an unprecedented high. There are several influencing factors that can lead to the development of insulin resistance including:

- An apple-shaped body (carrying more weight around the mid-section)
- Elevated triglycerides
- Elevated cholesterol levels
- Obesity
- High blood pressure

- Heart disease
- Family history of Type 2 diabetes
- Gestational diabetes (diabetes during pregnancy)
- Acanthosis nigricans (darkened patches of skin at the neck and sometimes the elbows, knees, armpits and knuckles)

Despite genetics or body shape, the main contributing reason that people develop insulin resistance is poor dietary choices.

The Effects of Insulin Resistance during Menopause

When a woman reaches menopause, it is almost like she is given a new body with a changed metabolism! The fluctuating hormones that are involved in creating this altered metabolism include the adrenal and thyroid hormones as well as progesterone, estrogen and testosterone. Considering that insulin is also a hormone that is greatly influenced by the other members of this close knit family of hormones, imbalances can very often occur in insulin during menopause. It is imperative to optimize the function of insulin before a balance can be achieved in the levels of estrogen, progesterone, testosterone, cortisol, DHEA and the thyroid hormones. For example, if you are experiencing hot flashes or night sweats, it will be very challenging to overcome these issues until the insulin has been balanced.

For many women, the apparent weight gain that often accompanies the onset of menopause is shockingly quick and immense. A common report of menopausal women is that they wake one day realizing they are suddenly ten to twenty pounds heavier with no obvious lifestyle change.

Menopausal women often experience fatigue along with the associated weight gain. Metabolism is compromised due to insulin resistance because the excess glucose in the blood stream has been converted into fat. Glucose receptors are found in high amounts in fat cells but due to the insulin resistance, the cells cannot absorb the glucose and this causes fatigue.

The cycle continues as a woman who is experiencing fatigue often will reach for foods dense in carbohydrates to boost energy which causes further weight gain.

Insulin Resistance Testing

Many people with fatigue, depression, hypoglycemia, excess weight or sugar cravings are suffering from issues dealing with blood sugar metabolism which is most often caused by poor dietary choices. Lab testing can help to determine if these issues are a result of insulin resistance.

The following items are included in the CardioMetabolic Profile from ZRT Laboratory:[41]

High Sensitivity C-Reactive Protein (hs-CRP)

C-reactive protein (CRP) is an established marker of inflammation and has recently been suggested to be an important contributor to pro-inflammatory and pro-thrombotic elements of cardiovascular disease risk. Overweight, obese, insulin resistant and diabetic individuals typically have elevated CRP levels.[42]

Fasting Insulin

High fasting insulin levels are a good indicator of insulin resistance which occurs when the cellular response to the presence of insulin is impaired which results in a reduced ability of tissues to take up glucose for energy production. Chronically high insulin levels are seen as the body attempts to normalize blood sugar levels.

---

[41] http://www.zrtlab.com/resources-and-data
[42] Marques-Vidal P, Mazoyer E, Bongard V, Gourdy P, Ruidavets JB, Drouet L,Ferrieres J. Prevalence of insulin resistance syndrome in southwestern France and its relationship with inflammatory and hemostatic markers. Diabetes Care 2002;25:1371-7.

Hemoglobin A1c (HbA1c)

HbA1c is a measure of red blood cell hemoglobin glycation. This indicates total and averaged glycemia over the previous three months which is the lifespan of circulating red blood cells. It can therefore indicate impaired glucose tolerance even when occasional fasting plasma glucose measurements are normal.[43]

Fasting Triglycerides

Hypertriglyeridemia, a triglyceride level >150 mg/dL, is an established indicator of atherogenic dyslipidemia and is often found in untreated DM2 and obesity.

Total Cholesterol, LDL Cholesterol, VLDL Cholesterol and HDL Cholesterol

Abnormalities in the lipid profile, including high total cholesterol, high LDL cholesterol, high VLDL cholesterol and low HDL cholesterol are significant components of coronary heart disease risk because of their contribution to the development of atherosclerosis.

Reversing Insulin Resistance

The function of insulin can be completely restored through proper dietary choices, targeted supplements and nutrients as well as consistent exercise.

The following foods should be eliminated or decreased significantly:

- Foods containing refined white flour and sugar such as breads, cereals, flour-based pastas, bagels and pastries
- Granola bars
- Protein bars
- Tropical fruits, fruit juice and dried fruits

---

[43] Geberhiwot T, Haddon A, Labib M. HbA1c predicts the likelihood of havingimpaired glucose tolerance in high-risk patients with normal fasting plasmaglucose. Ann Clin Biochem. 2005;42:193-5.

- All foods containing high-fructose corn syrup
- All processed or junk foods
- Condiments-teriyaki sauce, prepared salad dressings, soy sauce, chutney, BBQ sauce and marinades
- Jams, jellies, processed honey and maple syrup
- Peanuts
- Processed meats-luncheon meats, sausages and bacon
- Deep fried foods
- Protein powders with added sugars
- All artificial sweeteners
- Caffeine and specialty coffees
- Pop
- Starchy, high-glycemic cooked vegetables such as potatoes, corn and root vegetables
- Foods containing hydrogenated or partially hydrogenated oils
- Processed oils such as corn, safflower, sunflower, peanut and canola
- Fish contaminated with mercury and other heavy metals such as swordfish, tuna and shark
- Dairy
- Alcohol

Healthy nutritional choices that will reverse insulin resistance include the following:
- Choose clean, lean proteins such as organic chicken, turkey, bison, lamb, lean beef and cold water fish- salmon, sable, small halibut, herring and sardines
- Organic Omega-3 eggs
- Low glycemic vegetarian proteins- hemp hearts, chickpeas, lentils and a variety of beans
- Raw nuts-walnuts, almonds, pecans, cashews, pistachios and macadamia (do not exceed ¼ cup per day)

- Low glycemic fruits- apples, pears, peaches, apricots, nectarines, plums and all berries (Any fruit with a peel that cannot be eaten should be consumed in very limited amounts)
- Vegetables grown above ground should be eaten in abundance (with the exception of corn)
- Detoxifying vegetables such as the cruciferous family should be eaten daily (broccoli, kale, collards, Brussels sprouts, cauliflower, bok choy, Chinese cabbage and Chinese broccoli)
- Foods high in fiber will assist in blood sugar balancing. Choose ground flax seeds, chia seeds, legumes, nuts and seeds
- Garlic and onions are great additions as they serve to assist in detoxification and help to decrease inflammation
- Use fresh and dried herbs such as turmeric, basil, oregano, ginger and rosemary
- Use cinnamon in abundance as it is a powerful blood sugar balancer
- Use organic coconut oil for cooking as it helps to stabilize blood sugar
- Green tea and other herbal teas
- Filtered and sparkling water
- Unsweetened almond or coconut milk
- Plain- 0% Greek yogurt

One of the most important aspects of balancing and restoring blood sugar levels is to eat regularly. Skipping meals should be avoided at all times.

Meal Timing and Food Combinations:
- Eat something every 3-4 hours to keep insulin and glucose levels normal.
- Eat protein for breakfast every day such as whole omega-3 eggs, a vegan protein shake or nut butters.
- Eat small protein snacks in the morning and afternoon such as a handful of almonds.
- Do not eat within 3 hours of bedtime.

- Combine adequate protein, fats and whole-food carbohydrates at every meal or snack.
- Always be prepared by travelling with snack sizes of raw nuts and seeds.

Targeted Supplements to Reverse Insulin Resistance

Chromium has been widely studied for support of blood sugar metabolism. It decreases carbohydrate cravings and can increase lean-body mass in obese patients as well as enhancing the effect of other weight-loss strategies.

Dose- 200mcg per day

Omega 3 Fish Oils improve insulin sensitivity, lowers cholesterol and reduces inflammation.

Dose-1000mg-3000mg per day in divided doses

Alpha Lipoic Acid is a powerful antioxidant that can reduce blood sugar significantly. It also can be effective for diabetic nerve damage or neuropathy. Dose- 300mg -600mg per day

Biotin has been shown to re-sensitize insulin. Dose-2000mcg-4000mcg per day

Antioxidants such as Vitamin C and E are very important in helping to reduce and balance blood sugar levels.

Dose-Vitamin C-2000mg-5000mg per day. Dose Vitamin E-400IU-800IU per day

Cinnamon-the extract of Cinnamon is a powerful blood sugar stabilizer. Dose 500mg-1000mg per day

Fiber- supplementing with additional fiber in the form of ground flax seed, sun fiber, apple pectin, oat fiber and PGX fiber is a crucial aspect to balancing blood sugar. Dose-35mg per day

Balancing Blood Sugar with Exercise

According to Glen Gaessar, Ph.D., a professor of kinesiology at the University of Virginia, "Exercise is essential because muscle is the biggest tissue in the body, making up 30-40 percent of body mass. It's the major site of glucose (sugar) disposal. Inactive muscle is not as sensitive to insulin."[44]

Insulin has been shown to improve by 50% when regular exercise is occurring. Insulin becomes more efficient because exercise allows the cells to open and permits glucose to enter and be burned for fuel.

The foundation of exercise may consist of walking for 30 minutes daily. Other exercise may be included dependent upon fitness levels and the degree of insulin resistance.

Vigorous and sustained exercise may be needed to reverse severe insulin resistance. This would include 60 minutes of continual exercise 5 days per week. The desired goal is to work at 85 percent of your target heart rate. This can be determined by subtracting your age from 220 and multiplying that number by 0.85.

Strength training is also very beneficial to help maintain and build muscle. This will also improve your overall blood sugar and energy metabolism.

---

[44] http://susandopart.com/2010/06/are-your-weight-issues-tied-to-insulin-resistance/

Action Steps to Reverse Insulin Resistance

1. Get tested- Cardiometabolic testing will reveal the level of insulin resistance.
2. Avoid foods that cause insulin resistance- refined white flour products, sugar, high glycemic fruits, processed foods, artificial sweeteners, condiments, processed meats, deep fried foods and high starch foods *(see nutritional guidelines in the insulin resistance chapter for a detailed list)*.
3. Avoid pop, juice and sweetened drinks of any type.
4. Avoid alcohol and caffeine.
5. Consume blood sugar balancing foods such as clean, lean protein, omega-3 eggs, vegetables grown above ground, raw nuts and seeds, low glycemic fruits, coconut oil, low glycemic legumes, garlic and onions *(see nutritional guidelines in the insulin resistance chapter for a detailed list)*.
6. Use herbs like turmeric, cinnamon, ginger, rosemary, basil and oregano.
7. Eat a combination of protein, healthy fats and complex carbohydrates every 3-4 hours.
8. Balance blood sugar with chromium, alpha lipoic acid, omega-3 fish oils, biotin and antioxidants.
9. Consume additional fiber to balance blood sugar and decrease appetite with ground flax seeds, apple pectin, sun fiber, chia seeds, PGX fiber, oat fiber and psyllium.
10. Exercise regularly- walk at least 30 minutes per day and add in resistance as well as strength training.

Medications that Cause Weight Gain

Certain medications have been known to cause weight gain. The response is often individual as not everyone gains weight on these medications. However if you are experiencing unexplained weight gain and are taking any of these medications, then this might explain the cause. If this is the case, then refer back to your prescribing physician.

The following list outlines the most common medications that cause weight gain:[45]

Antidepressants
- Certain monoamine oxidase inhibitors, including phenelzine, isocarboxazid and tranylcypromine.
- Certain tricyclic antidepressants (TCAs). Tertiary TCAs including amitriptyline, imipramine and doxepin tend to cause the most weight gain. Secondary TCAs desipramine and nortriptyline may cause mild weight gain.
- Selective serotonin reuptake inhibitors (SSRIs) may less commonly cause weight gain (paroxetine in particular, in addition to fluoxetine or citalopram).
- Tetracyclic antidepressant mirtazapine

---

[45] http://www.doctoroz.com/article/medications-may-cause-weight-gain

Antipsychotics
- Many antipsychotics, including chlorpromazine, clozapine, fluphenazine, haloperidol, olanzapine, risperidone, sertindole, thioridazine, mesoridazine and rarely quetiapine.

Anticonvulsants/Mood Stabilizers
- Medications such as valproic acid, carbamazepine (rarely), lithium, gabapentin and vigabatrin.

Migraine Medications
- As mentioned in above categories, certain medications that are also used to treat migraines, like gabapentin, valproic acid, SSRIs and TCAs.

Beta Blockers
- Beta blockers including propranolol, atenolol and metoprolol which are used to treat a variety of cardiac issues may cause weight gain, possibly due to fluid retention or other factors.

Calcium Channel Blockers
- Flunarizine, which is not available in the USA One study suggested that verapamil may cause weight gain in some people as well. Anyone who rapidly gains weight after starting a calcium channel blocker should consult their doctor right away.

Alpha Agonist Anti-Hypertensive
- Clonidine rarely causes weight gain.

Diabetes Medications
- Insulin

- Most sulfonylurea medications including tolazamide and glipizide
- Non-sulfonylurea secretagogues repaglinide and nateglinide and thiazolidinediones like rosiglitazone or pioglitazone have been reported to cause weight gain.

Hormones

- Many studies have debunked the idea that birth control pills cause weight gain but they may cause a slight increase in water retention. However, medroxyprogesterone acetate (also known as Depo-Provera) or the etonogestrel implant, other forms of birth control, may cause weight gain.
- Megestrol acetate is a hormone sometimes used to stimulate appetite in cancer patients or other conditions that cause weight loss.
- Corticosteroids such as prednisone that are used to treat inflammatory conditions, especially if used long-term.

Cholesterol/Lipid-Lowering Drugs

- Clofibrate may cause slight weight gain but is not commonly used.

Antihistamines

- Chronic use of antihistamines such as loratadine, cyproheptadine, fexofenadine, cetirizine and diphenhydramine

Antiretrovirals

- Protease inhibitors often used to treat HIV including stavudine, zalcitabine, didanosine, lopinavir/ritonavir, indinavir, nelfinavir and saquinavir/ritonavir.

Cancer-Fighting Agents

- Cancer-fighting drugs cyclophosphamide, methotrexate and 5-fluorouracil, aromatase inhibitors and tamoxifen

Common Drugs That May Lead to Weight Gain[46]

Medication	Generic Name	Drug Class or Use
Paxil	Paroxetine	SSRI Antidepressant
Zoloft	Sertraline	SSRI Antidepressant
Elavil	Amitriptyline	Tricyclic Antidepressant
Remeron	Mirtazapine	Antidepressant
Clozaril	Clozapine	Antipsychotic/Mood Stabilizer
Zyprexa	Olanzapine	Antipsychotic/Mood Stabilizer
Risperdal	Risperidone	Antipsychotic/Mood Stabilizer
Seroquel	Quetiapine	Antipsychotic/Mood Stabilizer
Lithobid	Lithium	Mood Stabilizer
Depakene, Depakote	Valproic acid, divalproex	Seizure Disorder/Migraines/Mood Stabilizer
Neurontin	Gabapentin	Seizure Disorder
Tegretol	Carbamazepine	Seizure Disorder/Mood Disorder
Lopressor	Metoprolol	Antihypertensive-Beta Blocker (blood pressure)
Tenormin	Atenolol	Antihypertensive-Beta Blocker (blood pressure)
Inderal	Propranolol	Antihypertensive-Beta Blocker (blood pressure)
Norvasc	Amlodipine	Antihypertensive-Beta Blocker (blood pressure)
Catapres	Clonidine	Alpha-2 Adrenergic Agonist (blood pressure,

---

[46] Cheskin L. (June, 2011) Prescription drugs that can cause weight gain. John Hopkins Health Alert. Accessed November 18, 2012.
Drugs.com (March 2012) Prescription Meds Can Put on Unwanted Pounds. Accessed online November 18, 2012.

Actos	Pioglitazone	Thiazolidinediones (diabetes)
Avandia	Rosiglitazone	Thiazolidinediones (diabetes)
Amaryl	Glimepiride	Sulfonylureas (diabetes)
Novolog, Lantus, Humalog (various brands)	Insulin	Diabetes
Diabeta	Glyburide	Sulfonylureas (diabetes)
Glucotrol	Glipizide	Sulfonylureas (diabetes)
Deltasone, Medrol, Solu-Cortef	oral prednisone, oral methylprednisolone, hydrocortisone injectable	Corticosteroid
Allegra	fexofenadine	Antihistamines
Zyrtec	cetirizine	Antihistamines

Top Lab Tests to Uncover Hidden Road Blocks to Weight Loss and Optimal Health

For some people, achieving a health goal can seem impossible despite a person's best efforts. Hormones play a major role in healthy weight management for each and every person. Often along the way, other imbalances can develop as a result of chronic stress, poor nutrition, toxin overload and good old genetics! These imbalances can sometimes get in the way of optimal health. Uncovering these issues is the first step towards conquering the frustration of road blocks that can get in the way of reaching a healthy and sustainable weight. Lab testing can reveal the unidentified roadblocks that cause weight loss resistance. Listed below are the most valuable lab tests and profiles when it comes to uncovering the sources that prevent optimal weight loss. *(See appendix for recommended labs-testing which is available through Dr Cobi www.drcobi.com)*

Food Allergy Testing

Food Allergy Panel (ELISA/EIA IgG Panel) - The presence of antibodies in the blood to certain foods comes from deep within the immune system. Consuming allergenic foods on a regular basis results in escalating inflammation in the body which can result in weight gain. Blood testing for food allergies can reveal the hidden allergies that are contributing to obesity.

The premise behind this testing is that high circulating levels of IgG antibodies are correlated with clinical food allergy signs and symptoms. The ELISA/EIA test itself involves testing with food antigens by adding a patient's serum and looking for a classic antigen/antibody interaction. Testing reveals the level to which a person is reacting rather than just a yes or no result. Once the level of antibodies in a person's blood has increased above the normal threshold, delayed onset reactions are most likely occurring. Reactions can occur anywhere from thirty minutes to four days after the initial exposure.

Lab Testing for Candida

Blood Test for Candida

An immunoglobulin test measures the level of certain immunoglobulins or antibodies in the blood. Antibodies are proteins made by the immune system to fight antigens such as bacteria, viruses and toxins. IgA, IgG and IgM are frequently measured simultaneously. Evaluated together, they can give health care practitioners important information about immune system functioning, especially relating to infection or autoimmune disease.

Blood analysis under powerful microscopes can be used to find Candida antibodies. When Candida takes on its fungal form, the immune system responds by producing special antibodies to fight off the infection. A large concentration of these antibodies in the blood is an indication of a Candidiasis overgrowth.

Candida Immune Complexes tests measure Candida specific IgG immune complexes. Immunoglobulin G (IgG), the most abundant type of antibody, is found in all body fluids and protects against bacterial and viral infections.

Stool Analysis for Candida

The stool is directly analyzed for levels of yeast, pathogenic bacteria and friendly bacteria. Stool analysis tests diagnose Candidiasis through a laboratory examination of a stool sample. If the stool contains abnormally large amounts of Candida, then Candidiasis may be indicated.

A stool analysis can also look at other digestive markers for determining Candida levels such as:

- Levels of beneficial bacteria in the intestines
- pH levels in the stool
- Intestinal parasites, worms and single-celled organisms such as blastocystis hominis and amoeba
- SIgA which is the state of your gut immune system (a low SIgA can indicate low immunity or gut inflammation)
- Leaky gut syndrome

Urine Tartaric Acid Test

This test detects tartaric acid, a waste product of Candida yeast overgrowth. An elevated test means an overgrowth of Candida.

The Organic Acids Test (OAT)

The OAT provides an accurate evaluation of intestinal yeast and bacteria. Abnormally high levels of these microorganisms can be linked to behavior disorders, hyperactivity, movement disorders, fatigue and immune dysfunction. Many people with chronic illnesses and neurological disorders often excrete several abnormal organic acids. The cause of these high levels can include oral antibiotic use, high sugar diets, immune deficiencies and genetic factors.

Candida Urine Test

Secretory Immunoglobulin A (slgA) test and intestinal permeability test can be taken to assess the permeability of the gut wall (leaky gut syndrome). This is associated with the development of food sensitivities and Candida infections in addition to a build-up of potentially damaging toxins.

Breath Hydrogen Test

Bacterial dysbiosis results from the same causes as a Candida overgrowth. This is a test for bacterial overgrowth or intolerances to lactose, fructose or sucrose. The test measures the amount of hydrogen on a patient's breath within a specified amount of time after they have ingested a sugar solution. An elevated level of hydrogen indicates an overgrowth of bacteria in the small intestine. This test requires that you drink a solution of lactose, fructose, sucrose or glucose in water.

The Hormone Weight Gain Connection[47]

Hormones are key players in regulating weight, metabolism, blood sugar, insulin and when and where the body stores fat.

According to ZRT Laboratory, the following hormone imbalances are key contributors to weight gain:

Estrogen Dominance – estrogen/progesterone imbalance leads to weight gain in hips and thighs, water retention and low thyroid/metabolism

Androgen Deficiency – testosterone/DHEA imbalance leads to decreased lean muscle, low metabolic rate with increases in body fat and lowered metabolic rate

---

[47] http://www.zrtlab.com/zrt-specialty-profiles/weight-management-hp

Vitamin D3 Deficiency – leads to hyperinsulinemia and visceral fat

Thyroid Deficiency – elevated TSH is indicative of hypothyroidism, low metabolic rate, stalled weight loss and obesity

Insulin Resistance – elevated fasting insulin indicates insulin resistance which is a precursor of metabolic syndrome. Insulin resistance increases appetite, sugar cravings and belly fat as well as inhibiting thyroid and metabolism. When combined with elevated HbA1c (Hemoglobin A1C), it is predictive of type 2 diabetes.

The following diagram designed by ZRT laboratory summarizes the hormonal links to weight gain:[48]

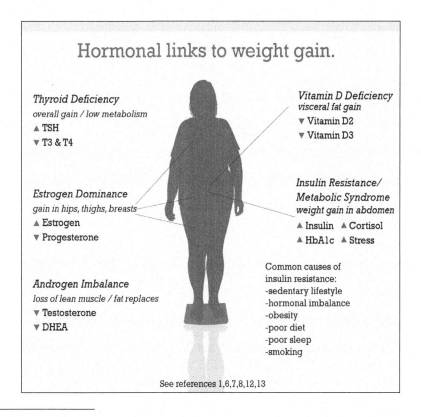

---

[48] http://www.zrtlab.com/zrt-specialty-profiles/weight-management-hp

Comprehensive Thyroid Panel

Imbalances of the thyroid are connected to many female hormone issues. These can include unwanted weight gain, breast cancer, uterine fibroids, ovarian cysts, endometriosis, infertility, postpartum depression, miscarriage, PMS and cycle abnormalities. Hypothyroidism or underactive thyroid is often linked with adrenal fatigue, estrogen dominance and progesterone deficiency. A dysfunctional thyroid can affect almost every aspect of health. It is one of the most under-diagnosed hormonal imbalances together with estrogen dominance and metabolic syndrome. A complete thyroid profile includes free T4, free T3, TSH and TPO which can indicate the presence of an imbalance in thyroid function. Hypothyroidism includes feeling cold all the time, low stamina, fatigue (particularly in the evening), anxiety, depression, low sex drive, weight gain and even elevated cholesterol levels.

The following hormones are included in the Complete Thyroid Hormone Panel from ZRT Laboratory:[49]

TSH – Thyroid Stimulating Hormone Produced by the pituitary, TSH acts on the thyroid gland to stimulate production of the thyroid hormones T4 and T3. Higher than normal TSH can indicate low thyroid function. Low TSH can indicate high thyroid function. Low TSH can also be caused by problems in the pituitary gland itself which result in insufficient TSH being produced to stimulate the thyroid (secondary hypothyroidism).

Free T4 – Thyroxine is the predominant hormone produced by the thyroid gland. It is an inactive hormone and it is converted to its active form, T3, within cells. Low TSH combined with low T4 levels indicates hypothyroidism, while low TSH and high T4 levels indicate hyperthyroidism. High TSH and low T4 indicate a thyroid gland disease such as autoimmune thyroiditis (Hashimoto's).

---

[49] http://www.zrtlab.com/resources-and-data

Free T3 – Triiodothyronine is the active thyroid hormone that regulates the metabolic activity of cells. Elevated T3 levels are seen in hyperthyroid patients but levels can be normal in hypothyroid patients because it does not represent the intracellular conversion of T4 to T3 which comprises about 60% of all T3 formed in tissues.

TPO (Thyroid Peroxidase Antibodies)

Thyroid peroxidase is an enzyme used by the thyroid gland in the manufacture of thyroid hormones. This is done by liberating iodine for the attachment to tyrosine residues on thyroglobulin. In patients with autoimmune thyroiditis (predominantly Hashimoto's disease), the body produces antibodies that attack the thyroid gland and elevated levels of these antibodies in the blood can diagnose this condition and indicate the extent of the disease.

Adrenal Stress Panel

The main function of the adrenal glands is to provide stress coping and survival responses. Higher and more prolonged levels of circulating cortisol like those associated with chronic stress have been shown to have negative effects on the body.

The panel utilizes four saliva samples. Salivary cortisol measurement reflects the free (bioactive) fraction of serum cortisol. The test report shows the awake diurnal cortisol rhythm generated in response to real-life stress.

The cortisol-to-DHEA (cortisol/DHEA) relationship highlights the many facets of stress maladaptation. The cortisol/DHEA ratio helps determine the projected time for recovery and the substances (hormones, supplements, botanicals) that promote this recovery. The cortisol/DHEA ratio regulates a multitude of functions.

The panel measures P17-OH levels in order to evaluate the efficiency of the conversion of adrenal precursors into cortisol. Certain adrenal fatigue patients who are genetically predisposed to low production of cortisol will not benefit from exogenous supplementation of pregnenolone or progesterone.

The panel includes fasting and non-fasting insulin measurements. The insulin values are used to diagnose insulin resistance-functional insulin deficit (pre-diabetes) as well as to correlate elevated cortisol with insulin to help explain glycemic dysregulation problems.

Total Salivary SIgA is included to determine the state of the immune system.

Gluten antibodies is included to determine the presence of a grain intolerance.

Female Hormone Panel

Dr. John Lee, the world's authority on natural hormone therapy, coined the phrase "estrogen dominance". This condition occurs when deficient, normal or excessive estrogen levels are not equally balanced with progesterone. Estrogen and progesterone work synergistically with each other to achieve and maintain hormonal balance in the body. The main cause of many hormonal issues is not the absolute deficiency of estrogen or progesterone but rather when estrogen dominates the hormonal pathway over progesterone. This domination of estrogen causes weight gain, especially around the midsection.

The following hormones are measured in the Comprehensive Female Profile from ZRT Laboratory:[50]

---

[50] http://www.zrtlab.com/resources-and-data

Estradiol and progesterone levels and their ratio are an index of estrogen/progesterone balance. An excess of estradiol, relative to progesterone, can explain many symptoms in reproductive age women.

Testosterone levels can also be either too high or too low. Testosterone in excess, often caused by ovarian cysts, leads to conditions such as excessive facial and body hair, acne, oily skin and hair. Polycystic ovarian syndrome (PCOS) is thought to be caused, in part, by insulin resistance. On the other hand, too little testosterone is often caused by excessive stress, medications, contraceptives and surgical removal of the ovaries. This leads to symptoms of androgen deficiency including loss of libido, thinning skin, vaginal dryness, loss of bone along with muscle mass, depression and memory lapses.

SHBG is a protein produced by the liver in response to exposure to any type of estrogen. SHBG gives a good index of the extent of the body's overall exposure to estrogens.

DHEA, mostly found in the circulation in its conjugated form, DHEA sulfate (DHEA-S), is a hormone produced by the adrenal glands and levels generally reflect adrenal gland function. It is a precursor for the production of estrogens and testosterone and is therefore normally present in greater quantities than all the other steroid hormones.

Cortisol levels indicate the function of the adrenal glands and exposure to stressors. Under normal circumstances, adrenal cortisol production shows a diurnal variation and is highest early in the morning, soon after waking and falls to lower levels in the evening. Normal cortisol production shows a healthy ability to respond to stress.

Free T4, free T3, TSH and TPO tests can indicate the presence of an imbalance in thyroid function which can cause a wide variety of symptoms. These symptoms may include feeling cold all the time, low stamina, fatigue (particularly in the evening), depression, low sex drive, weight gain and high cholesterol.

Male Hormone Panel

The following hormones are measured in the Comprehensive Female Profile from ZRT Laboratory:[51]

Estradiol is tested because too much of it, relative to testosterone levels, suppresses testosterone receptors in target tissues and eventually leads to feminizing effects in men such as breast enlargement. In healthy young men, testosterone is at its highest level and estradiol is very low. However, as men age, this shifts to a higher estradiol/testosterone ratio. Even if testosterone levels are normal, symptoms can indicate a functional testosterone deficiency because of the effects of higher than normal estradiol levels.

Testosterone is the primary indicator of male hypogonadism and andropause. Many things can contribute to low testosterone levels including high cortisol levels and high estrogen levels.

SHBG binds and transports both testosterone and estrogens in the bloodstream and it therefore regulates the relative amounts of free and bound hormone and consequently their bioavailability to target tissues. SHBG is a protein produced by the liver in response to exposure to any type of estrogen. Testosterone binds about three times more tightly to SHBG than estradiol. This increase in SHBG is a result of estrogen exposure which causes the relative proportion of bioavailable testosterone to estradiol to decrease even further, exacerbating the symptoms of testosterone deficiency.

---

[51] http://www.zrtlab.com/resources-and-data

PSA is a measure of prostate health and high levels can indicate the presence of BPH (Benign Prostate Hypertrophy) or advancing prostate cancer.

DHEA is a precursor for the production of estrogens and testosterone and is therefore normally present in greater quantities than all the other steroid hormones. It is mostly found in the circulation in its conjugated form, DHEA sulfate (DHEA-S). The production of DHEA occurs in the adrenal glands and declines gradually with age. Like cortisol, it is involved with immune function and a balance between the two is essential. Low DHEA can result in reduced libido and general malaise.

Cortisol levels indicate the function of the adrenal glands and exposure to stressors. Under normal circumstances, adrenal cortisol production shows a diurnal variation and is highest early in the morning soon after waking and falls to lower levels in the evening. Normal cortisol production shows a healthy ability to respond to stress.

Free T4, free T3, TSH and TPO tests can indicate the presence of an imbalance in thyroid function which can cause a wide variety of symptoms. These symptoms may include feeling cold all the time, low stamina, fatigue (particularly in the evening), depression, low sex drive, weight gain and high cholesterol.

Insulin Resistance Testing

Many people with fatigue, depression, hypoglycemia, excess weight or sugar cravings are suffering from issues dealing with blood sugar metabolism which is most often caused by poor dietary choices.

The following items are included in the CardioMetabolic Profile from ZRT Laboratory:[52]

---

[52] http://www.zrtlab.com/resources-and-data

High Sensitivity C-Reactive Protein (hs-CRP)

C-reactive protein (CRP) is an established marker of inflammation and has recently been suggested to be an important contributor to pro-inflammatory and pro-thrombotic elements of cardiovascular disease risk. Overweight, obese, insulin resistant and diabetic individuals typically have elevated CRP levels.[53]

Fasting Insulin

High fasting insulin levels are a good indicator of insulin resistance which occurs when the cellular response to the presence of insulin is impaired which results in a reduced ability of tissues to take up glucose for energy production. Chronically high insulin levels are seen as the body attempts to normalize blood sugar levels.

Hemoglobin A1c (HbA1c)

HbA1c is a measure of red blood cell hemoglobin glycation. This indicates total and averaged glycemia over the previous three months which is the lifespan of circulating red blood cells. It can therefore indicate impaired glucose tolerance even when occasional fasting plasma glucose measurements are normal.[54]

Fasting Triglycerides

Hypertriglyeridemia, a triglyceride level >150 mg/dL, is an established indicator of atherogenic dyslipidemia and is often found in untreated DM2 and obesity.

---

[53] Marques-Vidal P, Mazoyer E, Bongard V, Gourdy P, Ruidavets JB, Drouet L, Ferrieres J. Prevalence of insulin resistance syndrome in southwestern France and its relationship with inflammatory and hemostatic markers. Diabetes Care 2002;25:1371-7.

[54] Geberhiwot T, Haddon A, Labib M. HbA1c predicts the likelihood of havingimpaired glucose tolerance in high-risk patients with normal fasting plasmaglucose. Ann Clin Biochem. 2005;42:193-5.

Total Cholesterol, LDL Cholesterol, VLDL Cholesterol and HDL Cholesterol

Abnormalities in the lipid profile, including high total cholesterol, high LDL cholesterol, high VLDL cholesterol and low HDL cholesterol are a significant component of coronary heart disease risk because of their contribution to the development of atherosclerosis.

Supplements for Metabolic Health

Supporting the body's natural processes through supplementation can be of tremendous benefit. Foundational nutrients are needed to maintain general health, energy production, bone and muscle maintenance and immune function. The following chart illustrates the best choices to assist with specific health challenges that a person may face.

Foundational Supplements	Energy	Metabolism
Multi Vitamin (Women's or Men's Nutrients- for women/men over 40-Douglas Labs; Metabolic Nutrition- a powdered nutrient formula combining all vitamins, minerals and extra Vitamin D3 and B-complex- Restorative Formulations) **Vitamin D3/K2** (Essential for bone, muscle, skin, immune and cognitive health- Liquid Vitamin D3/K2-Thorne) **Omega 3's** (The purest and most potent Omega 3 fish oils- Klean Omega- Douglas Labs; EPA 720/EPA 500- Metagenics)	**Vitamin B-complex** (Great for stress, stamina, nervous system support and adrenal health- Stress B-Complex- Thorne; Multi B6-Thorne) **Vitamin B-12** (The most absorbable and active form of B12- Methylcobalamin 5mg/15mg-AOR) **Co Q-10** (The most absorbable form of Co Q-10- Q-Best 100mg-Thorne) **Iron** (The best iron for sensitive stomach's- Ferrasorb- Thorne)	**L-Carnitine** (Helps cells to burn fat, increase energy, improves heart and liver health. It also has the ability to reduce post exercise muscle damage, pain and tenderness) **Green Tea Extract** (Promotes the use of calories as energy and therefore assists our fat fighting efforts) **Garcinia Cambogia** (Inhibits the production of excess fat in the body as well as potentially suppressing appetite, making this a dual action fat buster)

Supplements for Metabolic Health

Calcium Magnesium (Cal Mag Citrate Powder- Thorne; Calcium Magnesium Capsules- Thorne) **Vitamin B-Complex** (The B vitamins are essential for proper functioning adrenal glands and nervous system- Stress B-Complex- Thorne; Multi B6-Thorne)	**Amino Acids** (An amazing powdered supplement that provides instant energy and enhances exercise ability- MitoVive- Metagenics) **MACA** (Great for energy, adrenal health and hormone balancing- Essential Ultra Maca- Dr Cobi; MACA- AOR)	**CLA** (An effective modulator of metabolism that is excellent for reducing stomach fat, increasing muscle mass and balancing blood sugar levels) **Green coffee bean extract** (Balances blood sugar in accelerates fat loss) **Raspberry ketones** (Decreases the absorption of dietary fats and inhibits the enzyme involved with starch breakdown and sugar absorption) (DL Weight Management Packs- Douglas Labs; Weight Release 1 and 2- Signature Supplements; Lipotrim- Integra; Xanthitrim- Douglas Labs)
Cravings	**Digestion**	**Stress**
L-Glutamine (This amino acid stops sugar cravings instantly. Take as needed or daily to prevent cravings- L-Glutamine powder- Thorne) **5-HTP** (Not only does this help with cravings but it also helps to decrease appetite and elevate mood- Brain Mood- Douglas Labs; Relaxeze- Enzed; Griffonia- Thorne) **L-Tyrosine** (The building block for adrenaline, thyroid hormone and dopamine which decreases cravings of all kinds including alcohol. Also decreases depression and improves mood so you are less	**Probiotics** (The "good" bacteria that are the foundation for optimal digestion- Ultra Flora Balance- Metagenics; HMF Intensive- Seroyal) **Digestive Enzymes** (Enzymes aid in the digestion of protein, carbs and fats. They greatly reduce gas and bloating and promote regularity- GI Digest- Douglas Labs; Ultrazyme- Douglas Labs; BPP- Thorne) **Fiber Formula** (Extra dietary fiber promotes regularity, detoxification, decreases appetite and balances blood sugar- Fiber Formula- Signature	**Relora** (Stress related eating over a prolonged period of time can lead to weight gain. This unique mixture of two herbal extracts is specifically designed to support normal mental functioning during stress and anxiety and normalize cortisol levels- Relora Plex- Douglas Labs, Relaxeze-Enzed) **5-HTP** (5-HTP is the building block of the "feel good" neurotransmitter Serotonin. It greatly elevates mood, balances appetite and helps to reduce stress- Brain Mood- Douglas Labs; Relaxeze- Enzed; Griffonia- Thorne)

likely to turn to sugar-Dopa Plus-Douglas Labs) **Chromium** (A simple trace mineral that balances blood sugar and prevents sugar cravings-Chromium- Thorne)	Supplements; Metafiber-Metagenics; Medibulk-Thorne)	**Vitamin B-Complex** (The B vitamins are essential for proper functioning adrenal glands and nervous system-Stress B-Complex- Thorne; Multi B6-Thorne)

(Items in brackets are Dr Cobi's top recommendations and are available on the online store at www.drcobi.com)

The Metabolic Plan

Now that you have discovered and conquered your roadblocks to weight loss, nutritional lifestyle changes need to take place. The Metabolic Plan is a 6 week plan to get you started. This plan should be maintained for life in order to achieve lasting and optimal health. Healthy nutrition is the fundamental reason that balance can be maintained in all areas of the body.

The Metabolic Plan includes the following:
- Organic Foods
- The Good, the Bad and the Ugly Fats
- Replacing Foods
- Tips for Dining Out
- Hydration
- The Maui Cleanse- Week 1
- The Metabolic Menu Plan- Weeks 2-6
- Recipes for Metabolic Health

Organic Foods

The Environmental Working Group has put together a list of the dirty dozen and the clean 15. This list refers respectively to the fruits and vegetables that are the most and least contaminated by pesticide use.

Pesticides are toxic to our bodies and different pesticides have been linked to a variety of health problems including hormone disruption, cancer and brain toxicity.

Switching to organic produce can be a gradual process for many people. Organic foods tend to be more expensive than their counterparts and therefore making informed choices in the produce aisle helps to minimize pesticide consumption while keeping the budget in check! When faced with the choice of a non-organic apple versus a bag of processed chips, remember that fresh fruits and vegetables, organic or not, are always a healthier choice than any processed foods. Processed foods contain a horrendous amount of chemicals as well. The following Dirty Dozen and Clean Fifteen chart is a guide to help you better allocate your organic and non-organic purchases.

The Dirty Dozen- Consume the 12 following fruits and veggies in their organic form as often as possible.

1. Peaches
2. Apples
3. Sweet Bell Peppers
4. Celery
5. Nectarines
6. Strawberries
7. Cherries
8. Kale
9. Lettuce

10. Imported Grapes
11. Carrots
12. Pears

The Clean Fifteen- no need to be organic!
1. Onions
2. Avocado
3. Frozen Sweet Corn
4. Pineapples
5. Mango
6. Asparagus
7. Frozen Sweet Peas
8. Kiwi
9. Cabbage
10. Eggplant
11. Papaya
12. Watermelon
13. Broccoli
14. Tomatoes
15. Sweet Potatoes and Grapefruit

The Good, the Bad and the Ugly- Fats

Not all fats are created equally and our bodies process and utilize fats based on their composition. Some fats are actually detrimental to our health while others can have therapeutic benefits such as decreasing inflammation, improving skin quality and increasing brain power. The following chart shows which fats to choose and which fats to ditch!

Great for Cooking	Great for Cold Uses	Good for Nothing!
• Coconut oil - Virgin, raw or unrefined 280°-365°, Refined 400°-450° • Butter (organic grass-fed)-325-375°F • Ghee (organic grass-fed) 425-480° F • Extra virgin cold pressed olive oil -320- 350°F • Avocado oil- 475°-520° (use sparingly and occasionally)	• Extra virgin cold pressed olive oil • Flaxseed oil • Avocado oil (use sparingly and occasionally due to its high fat content) • Nut oils (Macadamia, Walnut, Pecan) • Sesame oil	• Hydrogenated or partially hydrogenated oils/ margarines • Canola oil • Corn oil • Grapeseed oil • Soybean oil • Safflower oil • Sunflower oil • Vegetable oil • Rice bran oil

Replacing Foods

One of the best steps to take when improving nutrition is to start by removing poor choices and replacing them with healthy alternatives. The following chart highlights poor choices and offers a better and optimal choice in its place.

Poor Choice	Better Choice	Optimal Choice
Soy sauce (loaded with sodium, gluten and often MSG)	Wheat free tamari, Bragg's liquid Aminos	Coconut liquid Aminos
Cow milk (inflammatory and highly allergenic)	Unsweetened Almond or coconut milk	Unsweetened Almond or coconut milk
Sweetened cow yogurt (loaded with hidden sugar)	Unsweetened, plain organic 0% Greek Yogurt	Coconut yogurt, Kefir (if tolerable due to dairy content)
Boxed cereals (highly processed and sugar laden)	Steel cut gluten free oatmeal	Grain free granola (Assorted chopped nuts and coconut)

Protein Bars (often filled with processed ingredients)	Homemade protein bars	Raw nuts and seeds
Pasta made from grain flour (high in simple carbohydrates, gluten and nutrient void)	Spaghetti squash, zucchini noodles	Spaghetti squash, zucchini noodles
Breads, buns, crackers made from grain flour (high in simple carbohydrates and loaded with gluten)	Sprouted grain, gluten free options	Grain free (Coconut flour or almond meal alternatives)
Rice (turns to sugar in the body)	Quinoa, Buckwheat, Millet, Steel cut oats	Cauliflower rice
Highly processed sugar laden treats (high in processed ingredients and sugar)	Homemade treats (energy balls, power cookies)	Grain free, sugar free alternatives (coconut macaroons, coconut cookie bars, apple loaf, pumpkin spice cookies)
Condiments and marinades (high in sugar, sodium and often MSG)	Wheat free tamari, Bragg's liquid Aminos, Apple Cider Vinegar, Balsamic Vinegar, Herbs and Spices	Coconut liquid Aminos, Apple Cider Vinegar, Herbs and Spices
Processed meats	Natural chicken breasts, turkey breast, extra lean beef, wild non-farmed fish	Organic nitrate free meats, organic chicken and turkey, organic bison, organic grass fed lean beef, wild non-farmed fish

Tips for Dining out

Dining out can become a real issue for many people when it comes time to making the right choice. Being informed and prepared will help you to make a decision you can wake up the next day feeling happy about.

Choosing a Restaurant

- Avoid "all-you-can-eat" places. More diets go here to die than any other type of restaurant.
- Choose a place with a varied menu. It'll make it easier to find something healthy and to your taste.
- Don't decide to eat out on the spur of the moment, if possible. It's best to make plans and account for it during the rest of the day's menu planning.
- Any restaurant with a mascot or a drive thru is probably bad news.

Before you leave your house

- 1-2 hours before you leave for the restaurant have a small snack so you do not arrive starving and succumb to temptation.
- Preview the restaurant's menu online before you go and decide what you are going to have ahead of time.
- Make a reservation to avoid waiting times and to prevent hunger.

At the table

- Pass on the bread basket! Ask instead for raw veggies or a few olives instead.
- Order a water right away so you have something to sip on. Better yet order a sparkling water with a lemon or lime so you feel like you are having something special to drink.
- Either skip the appetizer or opt for a starter salad with a lemon wedge or vinaigrette dressing on the side.
- Do not feel pressured or rushed to make a split decision. If you need more time to figure it out then ask!
- Do not be afraid to ask for something that is not on the menu or to ask for substitutions. Often a group of side items can make a great meal.

The Main Event

- Look for grilled, broiled or baked options. Skip the breaded choices which are often deep fried.
- Skip the rice and ask for double veggies instead.
- Ask for sauces on the side.
- When faced with the only option of a burger, ask to have it without the bun or wrapped in lettuce.
- Substitute French fries for a garden salad or for raw or steamed veggies.

Party time

- Avoid awkward social settings by asking the host ahead of time what they plan on serving so you know what to expect.
- Make sure to bring a dish or two that you know you can eat in case they are serving foods that you are avoiding.
- Have a snack before you arrive to avoid over eating.

Hydration

Next to oxygen, water is the human body's most important nutrient. Yet 75% of North Americans are chronically dehydrated and fail to drink the recommended amount of water per day. Up to 60% of the human body is made up of water:

- Your muscles are 75% water
- Your brain cells are 85% water
- Your blood is 82% water
- Your bones are 25% water

Water plays a vital role in many processes in the body including:
- Regulating body temperature
- Transporting nutrients to cells
- Removing waste
- Cushioning joints
- Strengthening muscles
- Protecting organs and tissues
- Maximizing mental function

The thirst mechanism does not actually kick in until the body is in a state of mild dehydration. "Dry mouth" is actually one of the last signs of dehydration. Chronic dehydration can lead to many symptoms in the body and can give rise to a number of disease processes:

- Arthritis
- High Blood Pressure
- Digestive Problems
- Asthma
- Skin Conditions
- Headaches/Migraines
- Constipation
- Memory loss
- Unexplained aches and pains
- Fatigue
- Dizziness
- Failing kidney function

Water intake and fluid balance are among the least understood and most neglected areas of overall health and weight management. Water is very important to health and our bodies are continually attempting to maintain proper fluid and water balance. Consuming too little water can actually result in water retention. Increasing water intake will decrease water retention along with bloating and the added weight that accumulates.

At normal activity levels, people lose two to three cups of water a day in perspiration. But during an hour of vigorous exercise, people sweat out approximately a quart of water.

Here are a few tips to help you drink the amount of water you need:

- Keep a water bottle that measures fluid ounces at home or at your desk so that the counting is done for you. All you need to worry about is finishing the bottle between the time you wake up and the time you go to bed. If a 64-oz. bottle appears too much to tackle, try a 32-oz. or 16-oz. bottle and just remember to refill it throughout the day.
- Keep post-it notes on your refrigerator or desk reminding you to drink a glass of water.
- Create a buddy system with a family member, friend, or co-worker to make sure you are drinking your water.
- Add lemon, orange or lime slices to your water to give it flavor.
- Remember to take baby steps and gradually work up to your goal of half your weight in ounces. It's never too late to start—this is for your long-term health!

*Divide your weight in half and this is how many ounces you should drink!

The Ultimate Metabolic Plan

The Ultimate Metabolic Plan is a 6 week program designed to remove toxins, kick start and repair the metabolism as well create an opportunity for a complete lifestyle transformation. Beyond the 6 week program, the nutritional recommendations should be continued for life. The first week of the program is considered to be the dedicated detox week; however, the process of detoxification will be ongoing as food choices that cleanse the body are consistently recommended. At any time, the Maui Cleanse can be done for a minimum of 3 days and up to 30 days as needed.

The following chart outlines the process of the Ultimate Metabolic Plan:

Week 1	The Maui Cleanse *(see below for instructions)*
Week 2-6 and onward	The Metabolic Plan *(see below for instructions)*

During the Metabolic Plan, supplementing with certain nutrients and herbs can greatly benefit the process. Foundational supplements are recommended for everyone at all times. The additional supplements can be taken as needed. (*Detailed descriptions and product recommendations can be found in the Supplements for Metabolic Health section*).

The following chart outlines the top recommendations for each specific need:

Foundational Supplements	Multi Vitamin- taken once with each meal Vitamin D3- 2000-5000iu taken once per day Omega 3's- 1000mg taken two to three times daily Calcium/Magnesium- 500-1000mg taken daily in divided doses Vitamin B-Complex- 100mg taken two times per day with food
Blood Sugar Support *(Choose one)*	Chromium- 200mcg taken three times per day before meals Alpha Lipoic Acid- 300mg-600mg per day taken in divided doses Biotin- 2000mcg-4000mcg per day taken in divided doses
Digestive Support	Probiotics- 15 Billion-50 Billion taken once per day on an empty stomach Digestive Enzymes- taken three times per day with each meal L-Glutamine- 5g taken once per day
Sleep Support *(Choose one)*	Melatonin- 3-5mg taken once before bed GABA- 500mg taken once before bed 5-HTP- 100-300mg taken once before bed Relora- 300mg taken once before bed
Adrenal Support *(Start with one and add additional choices as needed)*	Ashwagandha- 100mg-200mg taken three times per day Rhodiola- 100mg-200mg taken three times per day Adrenal Cell Extracts-as directed because individual products vary in dosing Relora-250mg taken two to three times daily

Metabolism Support *(Start with one and add additional choices as needed)*	L-Carnitine-600mg per day taken in divided doses Green Tea Extract-200mg per day taken in divided doses Garcinia Cambogia- 400mg per day taken in divided doses Green Coffee Bean Extract-600mg per day taken in divided doses Raspberry Ketones-300mg per day taken in divided doses
Craving Support *(Start with one and add additional choices as needed)*	L-Tyrosine- 500mg taken three times per day before meals 5-HTP- 100mg taken three times per day before meals L-Glutamine- ¼ tsp. of powdered glutamine mixed with 1-2 ounces of water-swish in mouth for thirty seconds and swallow for instant craving reduction
Energy Support *(Start with one and add additional choices as needed)*	Co Q-10-100mg taken one to two times per day MACA- 750mg taken two times per day Vitamin B12- 1mg-5mg dissolved under the tongue once per day

The Maui Cleanse

The Maui Cleanse is the perfect cleanse to achieve fast and effective weight loss and detoxification results. The Metabolic Plan begins with the Maui Cleanse in order to rid the body of toxins and to jump start the metabolism. Detoxification and cleansing are essential components toward optimal health. The duration of this cleanse is 7 days. Many people feel overwhelmed at the thought of a cleanse. The Maui cleanse was designed to actually make life easier! During this cleanse, there is less food to prepare than normal because two meals per day are replaced with a detoxifying smoothie. Many patients report that they find the Maui Cleanse very easy and convenient. In fact, many people decide to stay on the cleanse for an extended period of time. There is no concern about feeling hungry during this process as many patients that have completed this cleanse have been grown men with big appetites!

Once completed, transition into the Metabolic Plan is the next step.

The Story Behind the Maui Cleanse

Several years ago, I was scheduled to go to Maui, Hawaii. I realized a few weeks before the trip that I desperately needed to go on a cleanse. My desire was to feel really healthy and energetic on my vacation so that I could fully enjoy my family holiday. I was dissatisfied with the cleansing programs on the market, so I designed a cleanse for myself. The results were amazing!

Shortly after I returned, I had several patients who were preparing for vacations and wanted to also do a cleanse before leaving. I told them about my success with the cleanse I had designed and so I recommended it for them. Patient after patient got the same results- weight loss, energy, improved digestion, clear skin and an overall sense of feeling calm. It quickly became known as "The Maui Cleanse" and it is now a standard part of my practice and is asked for by name from people all over the world!

During a cleanse it is not uncommon to experience temporary detox symptoms. The degree of symptoms depends of the level of toxicity in the body. Common detox symptoms may include headaches, muscle soreness, joint pain, fatigue, nausea, a change in bowel movements and flu-like symptoms. Many people do not experience these symptoms and feel fantastic and energized immediately.

The Basics of the Maui Cleanse:

Consume a meal replacement detoxification shake for breakfast and lunch. Dinner should include a protein source and a variety of vegetables. 1-2 snacks can be chosen from the Snack Option list as needed.

Supplements for the Maui Cleanse:

Pure Lean Detoxifying Protein Powder-Pure Encapsulations (or other low carb vegan protein powder)- 1 scoop 2 times per day

Detox Fiber Cleanse-Dr Cobi or Medibulk-Thorne or Metafiber-Metagenics (or other blood sugar balancing fiber powder)- 1 tbsp. added to each shake

DL Detox Nutrients-Douglas Labs 1-2 packages per day with dinner **or LVDTX-Douglas Labs or Liver Support RX-Restorative Formulations or LCH-Thorne**- 1 tablet 3 times per day with food

Consume the following foods during the cleanse:

Domestic Fruit -2-3 servings per day
- Apples, Peaches, Pears, Plums, Apricots, Berries (raspberry, strawberry, blueberry, cranberry) (1 cup berries=1 serving)

Veggies grown above ground –Unlimited
- Artichoke, Arugula, Asparagus, Avocado, Bamboo Shoots, Beet tops, Bok choy, Broccoli, Brussels sprouts, Cabbage – all types, **Carrots**, Cauliflower, Celery, Chives, Cucumber, Dandelion greens, Eggplant, Endive, **Garlic**, Green beans, Jicama, Kale, Kohlrabi, Leeks, Lettuce – red or green leaf and all types of greens, Okra, **Onions**, Peppers (all kinds), **Radish**, Red leaf chicory, Sea vegetables – seaweed, kelp, Nori, dulse, hiziki, Peas – all types, Spinach, Sprouts (*broccoli and bean), Squash, Swiss chard, Tomatoes, Watercress, Zucchini **(veggies in bold are grown below ground but still acceptable)**

Clean, lean protein –Organic is best
- Chicken, Turkey, Fish, Wild game, Lean beef, Eggs

Raw nuts and seeds- ¼ cup per day
- Almonds, Brazil nuts, Chia seeds, Cashews, Flax seeds, Hemp seeds Hazelnuts (Filberts), Macadamia nuts, Pecans, Pine nuts, Pumpkin seeds Sesame seeds, Sunflower seeds, Walnuts

Legumes- 1 cup cooked per day
- All beans, Lentils – brown, green, red, split peas – yellow, green (All the above beans can be bought dried or canned without added sugar)

All spices

Misc.
- Braggs Liquid Aminos, Coconut Liquid Aminos, Apple Cider Vinegar, Balsamic Vinegar, Red Wine Vinegar, Lemon and Lime juice, Stevia or Xylitol

Flours
- Coconut flour, Almond meal

Beverages
- Herbal tea, Green tea, Purified water, Sparkling water, Organic Coffee- 1 cup

Omega Oils
- Coconut oil, Flax seed, Extra Virgin Olive oil, Nut oils (Macadamia, Walnut, Pecan) and Sesame oil

Avoid at all times during the cleanse:

Dairy Products
- Butter, Milk, Cream, Ice cream, Sour cream, Whipped cream, Cow cheeses, Whey, Yogurt

All sugar
- Artificial sweeteners, Barley malt, Brown sugar, Coconut sap, Corn syrup, Granulated & powdered Sugar, Date sugar, Dextrose, Fructose, Glucose, Maple syrup, Mannitol, Molasses, Monosaccharides, Sorbitol, Sucralose, Sucrose, Turbinado sugar

All grains
- Rice, Quinoa, Millet, Amaranth, Barley, Rye, Kamut, Spelt, Teff, Tricicale, Oats, Tapioca, Buckwheat

All processed foods

Soy (except Braggs Liquid Aminos, Non-GMO tofu, Tempeh)

Pork

Veggies grown below ground (some exceptions- see above ground in bold)

Corn

Tropical fruits, Dried fruit

Beverages
- Fruit juice, Pop, Alcohol, Energy drinks, Diet drinks, Soy milk

Misc.
- White vinegar, Mustard, Ketchup, Worcestershire, BBQ sauce, Mayonnaise, Refined, cooked, hydrogenated, fractionated or super-heated vegetable oils

Breakfast Shake:

- Pure Lean Protein Powder (1 scoop)
- Fiber Cleanse or Medibulk or Metafiber (1 tbsp.)
- 6-8 oz. water OR unsweetened almond or coconut milk
- 1 cup fresh or frozen berries
- 1 handful fresh greens (kale, spinach, Swiss chard, beet greens etc.)

Optional additional items that can be added to shake:

- Chia seeds-1 tbsp.
- Hemp hearts- 1 tbsp.

- Ground flax seeds- 1 tbsp.
- Flax oil (1-2 tbsp.)

Snack Options:
- Raw veggies with salsa or ¼ cup hummus
- Domestic fruit with ¼ cup raw nuts and seeds
- Hard boiled eggs
- 2 oz. chicken with raw veggies
- 1 pc coconut bread toast with 1 tbsp. nut butter
- Paleo muffin (see recipes)

Dinner Options:
- Chicken breast with raw veggies and salsa or hummus
- Grilled white fish topped with lemon and dill with steamed veggies
- Egg white scramble- egg whites scrambled with veggies (asparagus, peppers, spinach, mushrooms, tomatoes)
- Non GMO organic tofu scramble- as above but replace eggs with tofu
- Chickpea stir-fry- chickpeas sautéed in coconut oil with veggies (grated carrots, peppers, zucchini, spinach, kale, tomatoes, green onions)
- Wild green salad with tuna
- Zoodles (Spiralized zucchini) with homemade meat or veggie sauce
- Tuna, grated carrot, green onions, chopped apple, chopped celery, lemon juice, apple cider vinegar, 1 tsp. organic mayonnaise and dill
- Grilled salmon with steamed or grilled veggies and cauliflower rice (grate cauliflower and sauté for 5 minutes in 1 tbsp. coconut or extra virgin olive oil- add spices as needed)

7 Day Meal Planner (*Items that appear in **bold** will have a corresponding recipe in the recipe section of the Maui Cleanse Recipe Category***)**

	Monday	Tuesday	Wed	Thursday	Friday	Saturday	Sunday
Breakfast	Detox Smoothie	Detox Smoothie	Detox Smoothie	Detox Smoothie	Detox Smoothie	Detox Smoothie	Detox Smoothie
Lunch	Detox Smoothie	Detox Smoothie	Detox Smoothie	Detox Smoothie	Detox Smoothie	Detox Smoothie	Detox Smoothie
Snack	Raw veggies with ¼ cup hummus	**Paleo muffin** (recipe)	3 stalks celery with nut butter	¼ cup raw nuts and seeds	2 hard-boiled eggs	Apple sliced with 1 tbsp. nut butter	1 pc coconut bread toasted with nut butter
Dinner	**Italian veggies with Artichoke hearts** (recipe) with grilled white fish (tilapia, halibut, cod) with lemon and dill	**Lemon herb chicken with zucchini relish** (recipe) and **lemony green beans** (recipe)	**Green Salad with Pumpkin seeds** (recipe) and Grilled Chicken breast	**Coconut ginger salmon** (recipe) with **steamed broccoli with herbs** (recipe)	**Turkey lettuce wraps** (recipe)	**Fragrant Lentil Soup** (recipe)	**Ginger Chicken Stir-fry** (recipe) with **Cauliflower rice** (recipe)

The Metabolic Menu Plan

The following meal plans have been created to make planning easier for you! Each day has the appropriate amount of protein, carbohydrates and good fats. Every morning, the day is started with a Breakfast shake so that adequate protein is consumed in the morning. Protein is needed first thing to turn on the metabolic processes and balance the blood sugar for the day. Breakfast substitutions can be made as long as there is enough protein in the substitution to fuel the day (see the Breakfast Alternatives list for ideas).

These meal plans are guidelines and you can use your own meal ideas as long as you follow the Food Lists. Additionally, the order of the meals can be swapped around as there is no set order to them. In other words, take them as they are or switch them up as you please.

The mid-day snack can be eaten in between breakfast and lunch instead of between lunch and dinner. A second shake can be consumed in the afternoon, if needed, on days of increased physical exercise.

Items that appear in bold (recipe) will have a corresponding recipe in the recipe section.

The recipes are divided into the following categories:
- Breakfast Smoothie
- Breakfast Alternatives
- Maui Cleanse Recipes

- Breakfast
- Soups and Stews
- Main Events
- Sides and Salads
- Baking and Sneaky Treats
- Dips, Dressings and Snacks

Items that appear in *italics* contain grains. For those who are following a Grain Free plan, substitutions have been made in the recipe or in the plan in brackets with GF for Grain Free.

Quick and Easy meal ideas have been added at the end for those days when the best of plans do not come together. It is important to have a handful of "go to "meals that you can prepare quickly to prevent poor nutritional decisions.

In addition, **Breakfast Alternatives** have been added for optional choices to the Breakfast Smoothie on occasion. The Smoothie is the best choice for optimal protein, nutrients and metabolic nutrition.

The Fundamentals of the Metabolic Plan

- Combine lean protein and vegetables at every meal.
- Eat when you're hungry. For some, eating 5 small meals a day will work well. For others, it may be better to have 3 main meals a day with one or two snacks.
- Limit your grains to 0-1 serving per day (2 servings if you're struggling).
- Limit your fruit to 2-3 servings per day of domestic fruit only.
- Consume adequate healthy fats every day.
- Drink 1 oz. of water per pound of body weight each day.
- Never miss a meal.

- Carry a cooler packed with your food if you're on the go. Don't use a busy schedule as an excuse not to eat properly.
- Eliminate processed, refined foods.
- Eliminate chemicals, preservatives and sugar (both real and artificial).
- Eliminate saturated and trans-fats.
- Eliminate juice, pop, sweetened beverages and sports drinks.
- Eliminate alcohol (another form of sugar).
- Eliminate all fast foods and convenience foods.
- Avoid most dairy products.
- Eat fresh foods (nothing from a box or package).
- Stick to proper portion sizes.
- Eliminate all baked goods *even gluten-free ones (breads, wraps, bagels, donuts, treats).
- Eliminate granola bars, fruit bars, and protein bars (some are just glorified chocolate bars).
- Don't eat breakfast bars & pre-made breakfast drinks (canned or in a carton).

In the following weeks, it is important to maintain this lifestyle change that you have embraced.

The following are the key points to help you to remain consistent so that you can continually move forward:

- Love yourself enough to have a priority to fitness. Schedule it into your day timer as an essential part of your life.
- Learn to recognize stressors before they become overwhelming. Take a monthly inventory of the ongoing stressors with an awareness and commitment to minimizing the effects through the appropriate action steps.
- Grasp the understanding that sleep is the one most important elements for achieving overall health. Without sleep, all other avenues of pursuing wellness are in vain.

- Water invigorates and vitalizes the human body in its entirety. It is crucial to hydrate the cells of the body so that they can function in the capacity for which they are specifically designed.
- Nutrition is the means of communication to the body that is either life giving or disease creating depending on your choices. Everything we eat is a biochemical message to our cells.
- Toxic exposure is extraordinarily high and the body requires detoxification on an ongoing basis.
- Supplements support the natural processes of the body and they are a vital component in the journey towards optimal health.

Foods to Avoid

Protein	Highly processed meats (bacon, jerky, deli meats, sausages, hot dogs, burger patties, frozen chicken fingers or nuggets) Pork Smoked & pickled meats Fatty cuts of pork, beef, chicken, or lamb Battered and fried fish Farmed fish Fast food Genetically modified soy products/tofu (ex. many tofu nuggets and veggie meats are highly processed and made with genetically modified soy)
Dairy	Cow milk Cow cheese Sweetened yogurt Cream Whipped cream Sour cream Whey protein Ice cream Butter (unless organic, grass-fed butter)
Nuts and Seeds	Peanuts (and peanut butters) Pistachios Any roasted salted nuts
Sweeteners	White & brown sugars Artificial sweeteners Barley malt Corn syrup/High fructose corn syrup Dextrose Fructose Glucose

	Mannitol Sorbitol Sucralose Sucrose Fruit bars, and protein bars Breakfast bars & pre-made breakfast drinks
Vegetables/Fruit	Genetically modified corn (choose only organic corn) Non-organic vegetables and fruit (Dirty Dozen) Canned vegetables and fruit Potatoes, fries, chips Corn flour tortilla chips Dried fruits Candied fruits Tropical fruits
Grains	Wheat White bread (eliminate all wheat breads for best results) White rice (including basmati and sushi rice) Cous Cous Packaged instant oatmeal Pasta White flour wraps Bagels of all kinds Donuts Processed crackers Pancakes, crepes, & waffles Granola bars Fast foods & take out foods (including pizza) Cold boxed cereal
Miscellaneous	Sauces & dressings (use olive oil, lemon juice, or balsamic vinegar dressing made from scratch) Condiments (mayonnaise, teriyaki sauce, soy sauce, etc.) Fried foods Convenience foods (frozen dinners, even if they say low calorie or low fat) Snack foods (chips, crisps, "100 calorie packaged snacks", dried fruit snacks, etc.) Pop, diet pop, sports drinks, energy drinks, sweetened beverages, fruit juices Alcohol Hydrogenated oils Corn oils, canola oil, soybean oil

Foods to Consume

Concentrated Protein	Serving size: 3-4 oz. cooked, or as indicated (1 serving = approximately 150 calories) Meat, poultry, and fish should be grilled, baked, or roasted; fish may also be poached Protein Powder- 2 scoops- Pure Lean/Vega lite/ Mediclear Eggs, 2 whole or 3 egg whites plus 1 whole egg Fish, shellfish, 3 oz. fresh or ¾ cup canned in water Chicken, turkey Lamb Beef, extra lean (5% or less fat); buffalo, venison, elk Organic Non GMO Tofu, 5-6 oz. or 1 cup (fresh), or 2-3 oz. cube (baked) Tempeh, 3 oz. or ½ cup – Seitan, 1/3 cup
Legumes	Serving size: 1/2 cup cooked, or as indicated (1 serving – approximately 110 calories) Beans – garbanzo, pinto, kidney, black, Lima, Cannellini, navy, mung, fat-free refried, green, non GMO Soybeans Bean soups, ¾ cup Hummus, ¼ cup Split peas, sweet green peas, lentils
Dairy/Dairy Alternatives	Serving size: 6 oz., or as indicated (1 serving = approximately 80 calories) Almond milk, plain unsweetened, 8 oz. Coconut milk, plain unsweetened, 6 oz. Goat mozzarella, part skim 2 oz. or ½ cup shredded Soft unripened goat cheese 3 oz. Goat feta cheese, 2 oz. Yogurt (Greek), plain unsweetened 0% ½ cup

Foods to Consume

Dairy/Dairy Alternatives	Serving size: 6 oz., or as indicated (1 serving = approximately 80 calories) Almond milk, plain unsweetened, 8 oz. Coconut milk, plain unsweetened, 6 oz. Goat mozzarella, part skim 2 oz. or ½ cup shredded Soft unripened goat cheese 3 oz. Goat feta cheese, 2 oz. Yogurt (Greek), plain unsweetened 0% ½ cup
Vegetables- Above Ground- Unlimited	Fresh juices made from these are allowed (1 serving = approximately 10-25 calories) Artichokes – Asparagus – Bamboo shoots Bean sprouts – Bell or other peppers Broccoli, Broccoflower – Brussels sprouts Cabbage (all types) – Cauliflower – Celery Chives – Cucumber Eggplant – Garlic – Green Beans Greens: bok choy, escarole, Swiss chard, kale, collards, spinach, dandelion, mustard and beet greens Leeks Lettuce/Mixed greens: romaine, red & green leaf, endive, spinach, arugula, radicchio, watercress, chicory Mushrooms – Okra – Onion – Radishes - Salsa (sugar-free), Scallions Sea Vegetables (kelp, etc.) Snow peas – Sprouts Squash: zucchini, yellow, summer, spaghetti Tomatoes or mixed vegetable juice (low sodium) Water chestnuts, 5 whole
Nuts and Seeds	Serving size as indicated (1 serving = approximately 100 calories) Almonds or hazelnuts, 10-12 whole nuts Coconut, unsweetened grated, 3 tbsp. Nut butter, 1 tbsp. Pine nuts, 2 tbsp. Pistachios, sunflower, pumpkin, or sesame seeds, 2 tbsp. Walnut or pecan halves, 7-8
Vegetables- Below Ground	Serving size: 1/2 cup, or as indicated (1 serving = approximately 80 calories) Beets, winter squash (acorn, butternut) Carrots, 1/2 cup cooked or 2 medium raw or 12 baby carrots Sweet potatoes or yams, 1/2 medium baked

Fruits	Serving size as indicated (1 serving = approximately 80 calories) Apple, 1 medium Apricots, 3 medium Avocado-1/4 medium Berries -1 cup Cherries, 15 Fresh Figs, 2 Grapefruit, 1 whole Grapes, 15 Honeydew melon, 1/4 small; Cantaloupe, 1/2 medium Nectarines, 2 small Orange, 1 large Peaches, 2 small Pear, 1 medium Plums, 2 small Tangerines, 2 small Watermelon, 2 cups
Grains	Serving size: 1/2 cup cooked, or as indicated (1 serving = approximately 75 – 100 calories) Basmati or other brown rice, wild rice Barley, buckwheat grouts, or millet Quinoa Teff Whole oats, raw, 1/3 cup; cooked oatmeal 3/4 cup Gluten free wrap (brown rice, Teff or millet), 1 wrap Low-carb tortillas, 2 small or 1 large
Oils-Good Fats	Serving size: 1 tsp. or as indicated Oils should be cold pressed (1 serving = approximately 40 calories) Flaxseed oil- 1 tsp. / Nut oil- 1 tsp. Cold pressed extra virgin Olive oil- 1tsp. Coconut oil- 1 tsp. / Avocado oil- 1tsp. Ghee (clarified butter)-1 tsp. Organic grass fed butter- 1 tsp.

The Metabolic Meal Plans

The following charts outline the Metabolic Meal Plans:

	Monday	Tuesday	Wednesday	Thursday	Friday	Saturday	Sunday
Brkfst	Breakfast Shake	Breakfast Shake	Breakfast Shake	Breakfast Shake	Breakfast Shake	Breakfast Shake	Breakfast Shake
Lunch	¾ cup black bean soup with raw veggies (celery, carrots, cucumber, peppers) with salsa dip	*Low carb gluten free wrap* with 2 tbsp. hummus, 4 oz. chicken, shredded carrot, peppers and a handful of wild greens *(GF-sub **Grain Free Wrap**)*	**1 cup veggie soup** (recipe), 12 Mary's Gluten Free Crackers and ¼ cup hummus *(GF- **Seed Crackers**- recipe)*	4 oz. chicken, raw veggies and hummus, 2 Kavli crisp bread *(GF-**Seed Crackers**- recipe)*	2 hard boiled eggs; cucumber and tomatoes in oregano, olive oil and lemon juice	**Coconut vegetable curry** (leftovers)	1 can water packed tuna, 1 ½ cups spinach leaves, grated carrot and cucumber slices, red pepper slices, 1 tbsp. balsamic vinaigrette
Snack	1 medium apple, 10 raw almonds	½ cup 0% Plain Greek yogurt with 8 walnuts crushed and cinnamon	1 hard-boiled egg with tomato slices	1 pear, 10 raw almonds	½ cup 0% Plain Greek yogurt with ½ chopped apple and cinnamon	Raw veggies and ¼ cup hummus	1 medium apple, 1 tbsp. almond butter
Dinner	Grilled chicken with ½ cup cooked quinoa and ½ cup roasted yams *(GF-sub **Cauliflower Celery Root Mash**)*	**Veggie soup** (recipe) with **wild greens salad** (recipe)	**Basic Grilled Chicken with orange spinach salad** (recipe)	Grilled salmon in lemon garlic and sea salt, steamed veggies (carrots, broccoli, cauliflower, peppers, etc.), baked yams in coconut oil	**Coconut vegetable curry** (recipe)	**Chicken Dijonaise** (recipe), **Sautéed Greens and Beans** (recipe)	**Turkey burgers** (recipe) with **Yam fries** (recipe)

The Ultimate Metabolic Plan©

	Monday	Tuesday	Wednesday	Thursday	Friday	Saturday	Sunday
Brkfst	Breakfast Shake	Breakfast Shake	Breakfast Shake	Breakfast Shake	Breakfast Shake	Breakfast Shake	Breakfast Shake
Lunch	**Lentil Soup** (recipe)	4 oz. chicken cubed, ½ cup quinoa, green onions, red peppers, tomatoes, 2 tbsp. ACV, 1 tbsp. Braggs, sea salt *(GF- sub 1 cup shredded cabbage)*	4 oz. chicken, wild greens, red peppers, tomatoes, cucumber, 2 tbsp. goat cheese, balsamic vinegar	**Chickpea Salad** (recipe) 2 Kavli crisp bread *(GF-sub* **Seed Crackers***)*	Tuscan Tuna Salad: 2 cups cannelli beans, 6 oz. tuna, ¼ cup chopped red onion, ¼ cup sliced black olives, 2 tbsp. red wine vinegar, serve over wild greens	3 egg whites plus 1 whole egg scrambled, 2 tbsp. salsa, 1 tbsp. 0% Greek yogurt, ¾ cup cooked black beans in low carb/Gluten free tortilla	*Low carb Gluten free salmon wrap*: 4 oz. salmon chopped, 2 tbsp. Greek yogurt, 3 tbsp. grated apple, ½ lemon squeezed, 2 stalks celery diced *(GF-sub* **Grain Free Wrap***)*
Snack	½ cup 0% Greek plain yogurt, ½ cup fresh berries, 1 tsp. honey (raw, unpasteurized)	1 apple, 2 oz. goat skim mozzarella cheese	1 hardboiled egg, 1 small apple or ½ medium apple	½ cup sliced strawberries, 1 tbsp. sunflower seeds, ½ cup 0% Greek plain yogurt	3 stalks celery with 2 tbsp. unsalted almond butter	Green Apple Salad: Chop green apple, red grapes, and walnuts sprinkled with a dressing made from honey, lemon juice and cinnamon	½ cup carrots sliced, ½ red pepper sliced, ¼ cup hummus
Dinner	**Sesame Garlic Chicken with tahini spinach and** *quinoa* (recipe) *(GF- sub* **Cauliflower Rice***)*	**Salmon Parcels** (recipe) **Twisted Asparagus** (recipe)	4 oz. broiled tilapia or other white fish with lemon, dill and parsley, **Steamed veggies/greens in coconut oil** (recipe)	**Ultimate Veggie Burger** (recipe) With **Spinach salad** (recipe)	**Chicken and Wild Rice Salad** (recipe) *(GF-sub* **Cauliflower Rice***)*	**Turkey Lettuce Wraps** (recipe)	**Curried Garbanzo Beans and Squash Stew** (recipe)

The Metabolic Meal Plans

	Monday	Tuesday	Wednesday	Thursday	Friday	Saturday	Sunday
Brkfst	Breakfast Shake	Breakfast Shake	Breakfast Shake	Breakfast Shake	Breakfast Shake	Breakfast Shake	Breakfast Shake
Lunch	1 cup cooked chick peas, 2 tbsp. diced red onion, ½ cup halved cherry tomatoes, ½ avocado diced, 1 cup chopped spinach, ½ lemon, sea salt	4 oz. chicken, diced butter lettuce or romaine leaves, 2 oz. grated goat mozzarella, 2 tbsp. salsa, chopped tomatoes, red onion	**Red Quinoa and Black Bean Salad** (recipe) (GF-sub 1 cup shredded cabbage and ½ cup shredded carrot)	¾ cup Sweet Potato Soup (recipe) 12 Mary's Gluten Free Crackers, ¼ cup hummus (GF-sub **Seed Crackers**)	4 oz. chicken, wild greens, chopped tomatoes, cucumber, red peppers, 2 oz. goat cheese crumbled, 2 tbsp. balsamic vinegar	**Protein Power Bowl** (recipe)	**Weekend Kale Salad** (recipe)
Snack	1 apple, 10 raw almonds	2 stalks celery, 8 baby carrots, ¼ cup hummus	2 hard-boiled eggs	6 cucumber slices, 4 red pepper slices, 1 stalk celery, ¼ cup salsa	1 apple, 2 oz. goat mozzarella	3 stalks celery, 1 tbsp. almond butter	¾ cup 0% Greek plain yogurt, ½ cup mixed berries, 1 tbsp. unswt. coconut, 1 tbsp. pumpkin seeds
Dinner	**Ginger Chicken Stir Fry** (recipe)	**Asian Salmon** (recipe) *Reserve some quinoa*	**Turkey Tacos** (recipe)	**5 Spice Chicken and Orange Salad** (recipe)	Tofu Scramble: 1 brick Non-GMO tofu, ½ cup yellow peppers, ½ cup red peppers, ½ cup diced mushrooms, ½ onion diced, 2 cloves garlic, ½ zucchini chopped, top with salsa	**Halibut with carrots and leeks** (recipe)	**Curried Chicken *Quinoa* Salad** (recipe) (GF-sub **Cauliflower Rice**)

The Ultimate Metabolic Plan©

	Monday	Tuesday	Wednesday	Thursday	Friday	Saturday	Sunday
Brkfst	Breakfast Shake	Breakfast Shake	Breakfast Shake	Breakfast Shake	Breakfast Shake	Breakfast Shake	Breakfast Shake
Lunch	1 can water pack tuna mixed with ½ cup grated carrot, ½ cup grated apple, ½ lemon squeezed, 2 tbsp. apple cider vinegar, 1 tbsp. dill weed and 1 tbsp. extra virgin olive oil 13 Mary's gluten free crackers *(GF-sub **Seed Crackers**)*	**Rainbow Collard Wraps** (recipe) with **turkey sausage** (recipe)	**Green salad with pumpkin seeds** (recipe) with 4 oz. chicken breast	Chickpea Salad 2 cups chickpeas 1 cup halved cherry tomatoes, 1 cup diced red peppers, 1 cup chopped cucumber, 1 tsp. Basil, 1 tsp. Parsley, ½ juice of a lemon and sea salt to taste	Wild Green Salad 2 cups wild greens, ½ med apple diced, ¼ cup diced celery, ½ cup grated carrot with 4 oz. salmon and 1 tbsp. balsamic vinaigrette	**Asparagus soup** (recipe) with raw celery and carrots and ¼ cup hummus	**Egg and grain free burrito** (recipe)
Snack	Raw veggies (Celery, cucumbers, tomatoes, peppers) with ¼ cup hummus	12 raw almonds 1 medium pear	12 Mary's Gluten Free Crackers, ¼ cup hummus *(GF-sub **Seed Crackers**)*	12 raw almonds 1 cup berries	**Raw energy ball** (Recipe)	1 medium apple sliced with 1 tbsp. almond butter	**Seed flat bread** (recipe)
Dinner	**Turkey sausages** (recipe)(save 1 for leftovers) with spinach salad- 2 cups spinach, ½ cup sliced strawberries, ¼ cup almond slivers and 1 tbsp. balsamic vinaigrette	**Italian veggies with Artichoke hearts** (recipe) with grilled white fish (tilapia, halibut, cod) with lemon and dill	**Saffron Lemon Chicken** (recipe) with **Mashed cauliflower** (recipe) and steamed asparagus	**Coconut ginger salmon** (recipe) With ½ cup cooked brown rice and **steamed broccoli with herbs** (recipe) *(GF-sub **Cauliflower Rice**)*	**Lemon herb chicken with zucchini relish** (recipe) and **lemony green beans** (recipe)	Pizza night! 1 coconut wrap or *gluten free wrap*- top with tomato paste and veggies of choice (peppers, zucchini, mushrooms, artichokes, olives, onions, spinach) and daiya cheese or goat mozza	**Coconut fried chicken** (recipe) with ½ cup baked sweet potato and grilled zucchini with extra virgin olive oil

The Metabolic Meal Plans

	Monday	Tuesday	Wednesday	Thursday	Friday	Saturday	Sunday
Brkfst	Breakfast Shake	Breakfast Shake	Breakfast Shake	Breakfast Shake	Breakfast Shake	Breakfast Shake	Breakfast Shake
Lunch	1 can water pack tuna mixed with ½ cup grated carrot, ½ cup grated apple, ½ lemon squeezed, 2 tbsp. apple cider vinegar, 1 tbsp. dill weed and 1 tbsp. extra virgin olive oil	Left-over Turkey and *Quinoa* Mix up *(GF-sub Cauliflower Rice)*	Left-over Meatloaf with raw veggies and ¼ cup hummus	4 oz. Chicken Spinach Salad (Grated carrot, Pumpkin seeds, ½ cup chopped tomatoes, ½ cup chopped Cucumbers, 2oz Goat cheese) Fresh squeezed lemon	Left-over Curried Chicken *Quinoa* Salad *(GF-sub Cauliflower Rice or Shredded Cabbage)*	Egg White Omelet with veggies (peppers, spinach, mushrooms, green onions) with raw tomato slices	**Green Apple Turkey Sausage** (recipe) ½ Avocado **Grain Less Veggie Cakes** (recipe)
Snack	12 raw almonds 1 medium apple	1 hard-boiled egg 1 medium pear	**Paleo Snack Muffin** (recipe)	Raw veggies (Celery, cucumbers, tomatoes, peppers), ¼ cup hummus	¼ cup 0% Plain Greek Yogurt 1 cup berries	1 medium apple sliced with 1 tbsp. almond butter	**Skinny Guacamole** (recipe) 12 Mary's gluten free crackers
Dinner	**Turkey and *Quinoa* Mix up** (recipe) *(GF-sub Cauliflower Rice)*	**Mini Mexi Meatloaves with mashed cauliflower** (recipe)	**Chicken with Asparagus and Almond Pesto Wild Green Salad** (recipe)	**Curried Chicken *Quinoa* Salad** (recipe*) (GF-sub Cauliflower Rice or Shredded Cabbage)*	**Fish n' Shrooms** (recipe) with Steamed Veggies: Broccoli, Cauliflower, Carrots	**Crock Pot Chicken and Veggie Soup** (recipe)	**Black Bean Sweet Potato Chili** (recipe)

Quick and Easy Meal Ideas:

- Chicken breast, raw veggies with salsa or hummus
- Grilled white fish topped with lemon and dill with steamed veggies
- Egg white scramble- egg whites scrambled with veggies (asparagus, peppers, spinach, mushrooms, tomatoes)
- Non GMO organic tofu scramble- as above but replace eggs with tofu
- Chickpea stir-fry- chickpeas sautéed in coconut oil with veggies (grated carrot, peppers, zucchini, spinach, kale, tomatoes, green onions)
- Wild green salad with tuna

- Green smoothie- Protein powder (Pure lean, Mediclear, Vega lite) with 1 cup berries, leafy greens (kale, Swiss chard, spinach), hemp hearts, ground flax, chia seeds, celery, cucumber and 6-8 ounces water

Breakfast Alternatives:
- 3 Egg white omelet with a variety of veggies (peppers, asparagus, mushrooms, zucchini, spinach, kale, onion, grated carrots)
- ¾ cup Organic steel cut gluten free oatmeal topped with 2 tbsp. chopped raw nuts and berries
- ¼ cup 0% Greek Yogurt topped with 1 cup fresh berries and 2 tbsp. chopped raw nuts.
- ¾ cup Quinoa Porridge (see Recipe)
- Coco Cakes (see Recipe)
- Grain Free Seed Pancakes (see Recipe)
- Almond Flour Pancakes (see Recipe)

Recipes for Metabolic Health

Maui Cleanse Recipes

Italian Veggies with Artichoke Hearts

Ingredients

- 1 tablespoon coconut oil
- 1/2 red onion, diced
- 1 zucchini, sliced
- 1 cup green beans, cut into 2 inch pieces
- 4 cups spinach leaves
- 1 cup artichoke hearts, halved
- 1/2 lemon, squeezed
- sea salt, to taste
- 1/4 teaspoon black pepper
- 1 teaspoon dried basil
- 1 teaspoon dried oregano

Preparation:

1. Heat the coconut oil in a sauté pan over medium heat.
2. Cook the onions for about 8 minutes on medium heat or until cooked through.
3. Add the green beans and zucchini and sauté about 5-8 minutes or until almost cooked.
4. Add the spinach and sauté another 5-8 minutes until cooked through.
5. Add the lemon juice, artichoke hearts, salt, pepper and herbs- heat through another 5 minutes.

Lemon Herb Chicken with Zucchini Relish

Ingredients

- 1 tablespoon coconut oil
- 1 pound chicken, breast or thighs, diced
- 1 lime, squeezed
- 1 tablespoon fresh marjoram, freshly chopped, or 1-2 tsp. dried
- 1/2 teaspoon sea salt
- 1/4 teaspoon black pepper
- 1 tablespoon coconut oil
- 1 red onion, diced
- 3 zucchinis, diced
- 1 tablespoon fresh oregano, freshly chopped, or 1-2 tsp. dried
- 1 lemon, squeezed
- sea salt, to taste; black pepper, to taste

Preparation:

1. Cut up chicken breasts and marinate in lime juice for 10 minutes. Heat coconut oil in a medium skillet to medium heat and cook the chicken with the lime juice (from marinade).

Sprinkle with marjoram and stir occasionally, cooking until no longer pink. Season with salt and pepper.

2. Meanwhile, sauté onions in a large skillet with coconut oil over medium heat until soft and translucent. Add zucchini and cook about 10 minutes, or until zucchini is soft. Add chopped oregano and lemon juice. Season with salt and pepper. Enjoy chicken with relish.

Lemony Green Beans

Ingredients
- 1 tablespoon coconut oil
- 1/2 tablespoon ginger root, freshly grated, or 1/2 tsp.
- dried
- 1-2 clove garlic, minced
- 1 pound green beans, stems removed
- 1 lemon, squeezed
- 1 teaspoon lemon zest
- 1 teaspoon dried basil
- Sea salt, to taste

Preparation:
1. In a cast iron skillet or nonstick pan, heat the coconut oil to medium-high heat. Add ginger and garlic and sauté briefly.
2. Add the green beans, lemon juice, zest and 1-2 Tbsp. of water and sauté/steam over medium heat for 10 minutes, stirring occasionally.
3. Add the salt and basil and continue cooking the beans until they are soft but not overcooked. Add a bit more water or oil if needed.

Green Salad with Pumpkin Seeds

Ingredients

- 12 ounces mixed salad greens
- 2 stalks celery, diced finely
- 1 cucumber, peeled and diced
- 1 cup sunflower sprouts, cut into 1 inch pieces
- 1 avocado, diced
- 1 cup raw pumpkin seeds, toasted on a pan
- 2 tablespoons apple cider vinegar or lemon juice
- 1/3 cup olive oil
- 2 dashes sea salt
- 1-2 dashes black pepper
- 1 teaspoon dried thyme
- 1 teaspoon Dijon mustard

Preparation:

1. Combine the salad greens, cucumber, celery, avocado and sprouts together in a salad bowl. Sprinkle the pumpkin seeds on top.
2. Mix the olive oil, apple cider vinegar, salt, pepper and thyme together in a small bowl. Add a little mustard if you are able to eat it to help emulsify the dressing. Otherwise, mix well and then drizzle over the salad.

Coconut Ginger Salmon

Ingredients

- 1/2 onion, diced
- 1 tablespoon coconut oil
- 1 tablespoon ginger root, grated
- 1/2 teaspoon ground fennel
- 1/2 teaspoon cinnamon
- 1 cup coconut milk
- 1 tablespoon lemon juice
- 1/2 tablespoon lemon zest
- 1/3 pound wild salmon
- 1/4 cup fresh cilantro, freshly chopped, or 1-2 tsp. dried
- Sea salt, to taste

Preparation:

1. Sauté the onion in the oil until onions are translucent, about 10 minutes. Add the ginger, spices and cook for another minute.
2. Add the coconut milk, lemon juice and zest- stir to combine. Place the whole fish fillet into the sauce and cook over low heat for about 7-10 minutes or until fish flakes away with a fork at the thickest part.
3. Garnish with chopped cilantro and salt to taste.

Steamed Broccoli with Herbs

Ingredients

- 1 pound broccoli florets
- 2 tablespoons coconut oil or olive oil
- 1/2 teaspoon sea salt
- 1 teaspoon dried chives
- 1 tablespoon fresh parsley

Preparation:

1. Steam or boil the broccoli florets until tender but still bright green, about 8-10 minutes. Transfer broccoli to a serving dish.
2. Combine the coconut oil or olive oil, salt, and herbs and drizzle over the broccoli.

Turkey Lettuce Wraps

Ingredients

- 1.5 lbs. extra lean ground turkey
- ½ tsp. garlic powder
- 1 tsp. cumin
- 1 tsp. salt
- 1 tsp. chilli powder
- 1 tsp. paprika
- 1/2 tsp. oregano
- 1/2 small onion, minced
- 1 bell pepper, minced
- 1 cup grated carrot

- 3/4 cup water
- 4 oz. can tomato sauce
- 8 large lettuce leaves from Iceberg lettuce

Preparation:

1. Brown turkey in a large skillet. When no longer pink add dry seasoning and mix well. Add onion, pepper, carrot, water and tomato sauce and cover. Simmer on low for about 20 minutes.
2. Wash and dry the lettuce. Place meat in the centre of leaf and top with tomatoes and salsa.

Fragrant Lentil Soup

Ingredients

- 1 tbsp. extra virgin olive oil
- 1 large chopped onion
- 4 cloves garlic, crushed
- 3 large carrots, diced
- 1 tbsp. dried thyme
- 1 tsp. garam masala
- 2 cups green lentils, rinsed and drained
- 8 cups water or vegetable stock
- 2 cups chopped tomatoes
- 4 cups baby spinach leaves
- 1 to 2 tsp. sea salt or Herbamare
- 2 tbsp. red wine vinegar

Preparation:

1. Heat olive oil in large pot over medium heat. Add chopped onion and sauté for about 5 minutes or until onion begins to get soft.
2. Add crushed garlic, diced carrots, dried thyme, and garam masala, sauté for another 5 to 7 minutes.
3. Add the lentils and water; cover pot and simmer for about 35 to 40 minutes.
4. Add chopped tomatoes, spinach, sea salt and red wine vinegar- simmer for another 10 minutes.

Ginger Chicken Stir-fry

Ingredients

- 12 oz. boneless, skinless chicken breasts (cut into bite sized pieces)
- 1 tbsp. extra virgin olive oil
- 1 clove garlic (minced)
- 1 tbsp. fresh ginger (chopped)
- 1 onion (cut into wedges)
- 1 red bell pepper (cut into strips)
- 1 c broccoli (cut into bite sized pieces)
- 1/2 c chicken stock (divided)
- 1 tsp. arrowroot powder
- 1 tbsp. tamari sauce
- 2 c cauliflower rice

Preparation:

1. Heat oil in large skillet or wok and add chicken. Cook for approximately 5 minutes. Remove and set aside.

2. Add garlic, ginger, onion, peppers, broccoli and 1/4 cup chicken stock to the skillet. Sauté for 5 minutes.
3. Meanwhile, mix the arrowroot powder into the remaining 1/4 cup chicken stock and tamari sauce.
4. Return chicken to skillet, add tamari mixture and boil. Stir until the sauce thickens.
5. Serve over cauliflower rice.

Cauliflower Rice

Ingredients
- 1 head cauliflower
- 1 tablespoon extra-virgin olive oil or safflower oil
- 1 medium onion, diced
- Coarse salt and coarsely-ground black pepper to taste
- Spices, herbs, and/or vegetables of your choice (see variation ideas below)

Preparation:
1. Wash and trim cauliflower
2. Grate cauliflower with cheese grater to rice like consistency. This can also be done in a food processor
3. Add olive oil to sauté pan along with onion. Sauté until softened.
4. If adding other vegetables, do so at this point and sauté.
5. Add cauliflower rice and sauté for 5-6 min so that it is still slightly crunchy.

Paleo Snack Muffin

Ingredients

- 2 1/2 cups almond flour
- 1/2 tsp. baking soda
- 1/2 tsp. salt
- 2 tsp. Xylitol or equivalent Stevia
- 3 eggs
- 1 cup fresh or frozen berries or chopped domestic fruit

Preparation:

1. Preheat oven to 300°F.
2. Use baking cups to line a muffin tin.
3. In a bowl, mix the dry ingredients and set aside.
4. In another bowl, mix the eggs, sweetener and pour into the dry ingredients. Mix well. Add the fruit and mix well.
5. Using a spoon, place the batter into the baking cups and place in the oven for 25 to 30 minutes. A toothpick inserted into the muffin should come out clean and the tops should be browned.

The Metabolic Plan Recipes

Breakfast

Breakfast Shake

Ingredients

- Protein choices: Pure Lean (1 scoop); Mediclear/Mediclear Plus (1-2 scoops); Vegalite (1 scoop)
- 1 cup fresh or frozen berries
- 1 handful raw greens (Spinach, Kale, Swiss Chard, Beet greens)
- 6-8 oz. water or Unsweetened almond or coconut milk

Optional additional items that can be added to shake:

- Chia seeds-1 Tbsp.
- Hemp hearts- 1 Tbsp.
- Ground flax seeds- 1 Tbsp.
- Flax oil (1-2 Tbsp.)

Egg and Grain-Free Breakfast Burrito

- 1/2 tbsp. coconut oil
- 1/2 onion
- 1 cup zucchini, sliced
- 3 cups spinach leaves, washed and chopped
- 1 lb. ground turkey
- 1 tsp. dried oregano
- 1 tsp. cumin
- 1/4 cup fresh cilantro, chopped, or 1-2 tsp. dried
- 1/2 tsp. Himalayan sea salt
- 1/4 tsp. black pepper
- 8 whole cabbage leaves, washed

Preparation:

1. Steam entire cabbage head for 20-30 minutes. Check cabbage after 15 minutes and take off outer leaves that are cooked. Cook cabbage until cooked through. Remove from heat and peel off the cabbage leaves when cool to touch. Use for burrito or sandwich wraps.
2. Sauté the onion in the coconut oil over medium heat until soft and translucent, about 5-8 minutes.
3. Add the zucchini, ground turkey, spinach, oregano and cumin. Cook, stirring occasionally to break up the turkey, until the meat is cooked through. Add the salt and pepper to taste.
4. Garnish with fresh cilantro if you have it on hand. Enjoy in a steamed cabbage leaf or raw lettuce leaf to make a burrito.

Turkey Sausages

Ingredients

- 1 1/3 lb. ground turkey
- 1/2 tsp. ground ginger
- 1 tsp. Himalayan sea salt
- 1 tsp. ground sage
- 1 tsp. black pepper
- 1 tbsp. coconut oil

Preparation:

1. In a large bowl, mix the ground turkey, ginger, salt, sage, and black pepper until well blended.
2. Heat a skillet over medium-high heat and coat with coconut oil. Form the turkey sausage into patties and fry until browned on both sides and no longer pink in the centre. This should take about 10-15 minutes depending upon size of patties. You can make 5-6 large ones or up to 10 small ones.

Green Apple Turkey Sausages

Ingredients

- 1 lb. ground turkey
- ½ green apple, peeled and diced
- 2 cloves garlic, minced
- 2 tbsp. onion, minced
- 1 tsp. Himalayan sea salt
- ¼ tsp. black Pepper
- 1 tbsp. sage

- 2 tsp. parsley
- 1 tsp. coconut oil

Preparation:

1. Combine ground turkey, apple, garlic, onion and spices in a medium sized mixing bowl.
2. Form the mixture into 8 evenly sized patties.
3. Heat coconut oil in a large skillet over medium heat. Cook the patties for 5 to 6 minutes on each side until cooked through and browned.

Grain less Veggie Cakes

Ingredients

- 3 cups grated zucchini
- 1 cup grated carrots
- 1 clove garlic, minced
- 2 tbsp. coconut flour
- ¼ cup coconut oil
- Himalayan sea salt and black pepper to taste
- 3 eggs, beaten

Preparation:

1. Squeeze the excess water out of grated carrot and zucchini using a piece of cheese cloth or paper towel.
2. Combine the eggs, garlic, salt and pepper in a large mixing bowl. Slowly sift in coconut flour and mix. Stir in the grated veggies.

3. Heat the coconut oil in a large skillet over medium heat. Add ¼ cup of the veggie mixture into skillet and cook for approximately 3 minutes on each side.
4. Allow to cool for a firmer texture or eat when warm.

Quinoa Porridge

Ingredients
- ½ cup quinoa, rinsed
- 1 cup water
- ½ cup quinoa flakes
- ½ cup chopped domestic fruit (Apples, pears, peaches, berries)
- Stevia or Xylitol to taste
- ¼ cup chopped walnuts

Preparation:
1. Bring the quinoa and water to a boil. Reduce the heat, cover and simmer about 10 minutes, until cooked.
2. Add the quinoa flakes, fruit, nuts and sweetener. Stir and continue simmering for another 10 to 15 minutes. The mixture should have a fluffy consistency.

Coco Cakes

Ingredients
- 4 eggs
- ¼ cup coconut flour
- ¼ tsp. nutmeg
- ½ tsp. cinnamon

Topping

- 3 tsp. water
- 2 cups domestic fruit, mashed with a potato masher
- 2 tbsp. arrowroot
- ½ tsp. Stevia or 1 tsp. Xylitol
- ¼ tsp. cinnamon
- ¼ cup coconut milk

Preparation:

1. Mix these ingredients and let them sit for five minutes. Melt coconut oil in sauté pan. Pour about a ¼ cup of batter for each cake, allowing each side to brown before flipping it.
2. For the topping put the water, cinnamon, fruit, arrowroot sweetener in a saucepan and bring to a boil. Turn down the heat and simmer for 5 minutes until the sauce reduces and thickens.

Almond Flour Pancakes and Waffles

Ingredients

- 1 cup almond flour
- 1/4 tsp. Himalayan sea salt
- 1/4 tsp. aluminium free baking soda
- 4 eggs
- 1 tbsp. Xylitol or ½ tsp. Stevia
- 1 tbsp. Coconut oil for cooking

Preparation:

1. In a bowl, mix the dry ingredients and set aside.

2. In another bowl, whisk the eggs and add them to the dry mix. Adding more flour will thicken the mix, if desired.
3. Melt coconut oil in frying pan and spoon enough mixture to make medallion sized pancakes.

Grain Free Seed Pancakes

Ingredients
- 1 cup raw pumpkin seeds
- 1 tbsp. whole anise seeds
- 2 tbsp. whole flax seeds
- ¼ cup arrowroot
- 1 cup warm water
- 1 tbsp. extra virgin olive oil
- ¼ tsp. Himalayan sea salt
- ¼ cup water

Preparation:
1. In a large bowl, mix the pumpkin, anise, flax seed and arrowroot- mix well with a whisk.
2. Take ½ cup of the mix and blend it in a blender on high for approximately 30 seconds. Using a spatula, move the mix from the bottom of the blender to prevent sticking and then continue blending for another 30 minutes. Mix should be very fine. Put in separate bowl and continue blending the rest of the mix in ½ cup portions until all the mix has been blended fine.
3. Add the water, oil and salt and the ground mix to the blender and blend again. Pour the mix into a large bowl and let stand for 10 to 15 minutes. (If you want to prepare this the evening before, you can let it rest overnight so it will be ready for breakfast the next day).

4. Heat oil in frying pan and then spoon the mix into the pan. You can prepare a double batch and freeze them for later use.

Soups and Stews

Veggie Soup

Ingredients
- 4 carrots, chopped
- 3 onions, chopped
- 2 parsnips, chopped
- 2 stalks of celery, chopped
- 4 tbsp. extra virgin olive oil
- 2 litres veggie stock
- 1 cup brown rice or millet *(GF-2 cups grated cauliflower)*
- 1 tsp. Himalayan sea salt
- 1/2 lb beet greens
- 1 cup cooked chickpeas, rinsed
- 2 tbsp. chopped parsley

Preparation:
1. In a large pot, sauté chopped veggies in oil until lightly cooked.
2. Add stock. Stir in brown rice, millet or grated cauliflower and add salt.
3. Simmer at least one hour or until barley in tender.
4. During last 15 minutes of cooking, add chickpeas and beet greens. Garnish with parsley.

Fragrant Lentil Soup

Ingredients

- 1 tbsp. extra virgin olive oil
- 1 large chopped onion
- 4 cloves garlic, crushed
- 3 large carrots, diced
- 1 tbsp. dried thyme
- 1 tsp. garam masala
- 2 cups green lentils, rinsed and drained
- 8 cups water or vegetable stock
- 2 cups chopped tomatoes
- 4 cups baby spinach leaves
- 1 to 2 tsp. Himalayan sea salt or Herbamare
- 2 tbsp. red wine vinegar

Preparation:

1. Heat olive oil in large pot over medium heat. Add chopped onion and sauté for about 5 minutes or until onion begins to get soft.
2. Add crushed garlic, diced carrots, dried thyme, and garam masala, sauté for another 5 to 7 minutes.
3. Add the lentils and water; cover pot and simmer for about 35 to 40 minutes.
4. Add chopped tomatoes, spinach, sea salt, and red wine vinegar and simmer for another 10 minutes.

Sweet Potato Soup

Ingredients

- 5 medium sweet potatoes, peeled and chopped
- 5 small organic potatoes, peeled and chopped
- 4-5 organic carrots chopped
- 1 onion, chopped
- 3 garlic grated or minced
- 1 tbsp. coconut oil
- 1 tbsp. extra virgin olive oil
- 1 can organic coconut milk
- Himalayan sea salt and black pepper to taste
- 3-4 tbsp. or more curry powder
- 1 tbsp. paprika
- 1 tsp. garlic powder

Preparation:

1. Sauté onion and garlic in 1 tbsp. coconut oil and 1 tbsp. olive oil for about 3-4 min. Add carrots, sweet potato, potato. Then add enough water to cover vegetables. Let simmer until vegetables are nice and soft.
2. Blend with hand blender, Vitamix or food processor until fairly smooth. Add garlic powder, curry powder and paprika- blend until completely smooth.
3. Stir in coconut milk, salt and pepper.
4. Adjust consistency by adding more water if needed.

Thai Coconut Vegetable Soup

Ingredients

- 2 cups vegetable or chicken stock
- 1 can coconut milk
- 1 tsp. crushed red chili flakes
- 6 to 8 cloves garlic, crushed
- 1 small onion, cut into half moons
- 2 to 3 carrots, peeled and cut into matchsticks
- 1 red bell pepper, cut into strips
- 1 medium zucchini, cut in half lengthwise then sliced
- 2 cups thinly sliced bok choy leaves or cabbage leaves
- ½ cup chopped cilantro
- Himalayan Sea salt or Herbamare, to taste

Preparation:

1. Place the vegetable or chicken stock into 4 quart pot.
2. Add the coconut milk, red chili flakes, crushed garlic, onion, carrots and red bell pepper. Simmer for 15 minutes, covered, or until the vegetables are just tender.
3. Add the zucchini and simmer 5 minutes more.
4. Remove pot from heat and add the sliced bok choy leaves, cilantro and salt.
5. Garnish with extra red chili flakes if desired.

Coconut Vegetable Curry with Chickpeas

Ingredients

- 2 tbsp. virgin coconut oil or extra virgin olive oil
- 1 tbsp. finely chopped fresh ginger
- 1 ½ tsp. cumin seeds
- 3 small red potatoes, cut into cubes
- 3 medium carrots, diced
- ½ tsp. turmeric
- 2 tsp. coriander
- 1 tsp. curry powder
- 1 tbsp. tomato paste
- 1 can coconut milk
- ¼ to ½ cup water
- 2 small zucchini, diced
- 2 cups cooked chickpeas (garbanzo beans), rinsed
- 2 tsp. Himalayan sea salt
- ½ cup cilantro

Preparation:

1. In a large pot, heat olive oil over medium heat. Add ginger, cumin seeds and cook for 1 to 2 minutes or until the seeds begin to "pop".
2. Add potatoes, carrots, turmeric, coriander and curry powder. Stir well and continue to cook for another minute or so. Add the tomato paste, coconut milk, water and stir well.
3. Simmer, covered, for 5 to 10 minutes until potatoes and carrots are almost done but still a little crisp. Add zucchini, chickpeas, and sea salt; cover the pot and simmer until vegetables are tender, about another 6 to 7 minutes. Remove from heat and stir in chopped cilantro.

Curried Garbanzo Bean and Squash Stew

Ingredients

- 2 tbsp. virgin coconut oil or extra virgin olive oil
- 1 medium onion, chopped
- 4 to 5 cloves garlic, crushed
- 2 tsp. curry powder
- 1 tsp. ground cumin
- 1 tsp. ground coriander
- ½ tsp. turmeric
- ½ tsp. cinnamon
- Pinch cayenne pepper
- 2 delicata squash, peeled, seeded and cut into chunks
- 2 cups diced tomatoes, or one 14 ounce can
- 3 to 4 cups chopped kale or spinach
- 3 cups cooked garbanzo beans, or 2 cans, rinsed
- 1 cup water
- 1 to 2 tsp. Himalayan sea salt or Herbamare

Preparation:

1. Heat an 11 inch skillet or 6 quart pot over medium heat. Add coconut oil then onions; sauté for about 15 minutes or until soft. Then add the crushed garlic and spices; sauté for a minute more.
2. Next add the delicate squash and tomatoes. Place lid on the pot and simmer over low to medium-low heat until squash is tender, about 15 minutes.

3. Then add the chopped kale, cooked garbanzo beans, bean cooking liquid, and sea salt; gently stir together and simmer for an additional 5 minutes. Taste and add more salt and seasoning if desired.

Asparagus Soup

Ingredients
- 1 pound asparagus
- 4 cups chicken or veggie stock
- 1 ½ cups spinach
- ½ cup fresh dill, basil or parsley
- ¼ tsp. nutmeg
- 1 tbsp. lemon juice
- ½ tsp. Himalayan sea salt
- ¼ tsp. black pepper

Preparation:
1. Trim the ends from the asparagus and cut into 1" pieces.
2. Place the broth and pieces of asparagus in a large pot and bring to a boil. Reduce the heat and simmer, covered, for 20 minutes.
3. Add the spinach, dill (or other herb), lemon juice and nutmeg, and simmer uncovered for 5 minutes. Season with salt and pepper.
4. Either using a hand blender, or transferring soup in batches to a blender, puree until well blended. Taste and adjust seasonings.

Main Events

Vegetable Jalfrezi

Ingredients
- 1 medium onion, chopped
- 2 inch piece of fresh root ginger, peel and finely slice
- 2 cloves garlic, finely chopped
- 1 small bunch of cilantro, chopped
- 2 red bell peppers, roughly chopped
- 1 cauliflower, broken into florets
- 3 ripe tomatoes, quartered
- 1 small butternut squash, peeled, cleaned and sliced into 1 inch wedges
- 1 15 oz. can of garbanzo beans, drained
- 2 tbsp. extra virgin olive oil
- 1/2 cup Jalfrezi or medium curry paste
- 2 14 oz. cans of diced tomatoes
- 1/4 cup balsamic vinegar
- 1 lemon
- 1 cup 0% plain Balkan style yogurt (optional)
- 3-4 cups brown rice (optional)

Preparation:
1. Heat a large pot on medium high heat and add 2 tbsp. olive oil.
2. Add the onions, ginger, garlic and cilantro until golden, about 10 minutes.
3. Add the peppers, squash, beans and Jalfrezi paste. Stir to coat.
4. Add the cauliflower, fresh and canned tomatoes and the vinegar.

5. Pour 1 1/2 cups water into pan, stir again and bring to a boil.
6. Cover, reduce heat and simmer for about 45 minutes. Checking to make occasionally. If too much liquid, leave lid off for the last 15 minutes.
7. Salt and pepper to taste and squeeze lemon on top.
8. If desired, serve over rice and with a dollop of yogurt (optional)

Ultimate Veggie Burger

Ingredients
- 1/2 cup onion, diced
- 1 large garlic clove, minced
- Flax eggs: 2.5 tbsp ground flax + 1/2 cup warm water, mixed in bowl
- 2 cups Gluten Free bread crumbs (GF-sub coconut bread crumbs)
- 1 cup grated carrots
- 1 cup cooked black beans, rinsed and roughly pureed or mashed
- Heaping 1/4 cup finely chopped parsley
- 1/3 cup almonds, chopped
- 1/2 cup sunflower seeds
- 1 tbsp. Extra Virgin Olive Oil
- 1.5 tsp. chili powder
- 1 tsp. cumin
- 1 tsp. oregano
- Himalayan sea salt and black pepper, to taste

Preparation:

1. Preheat oven to 350F (if baking). In a large skillet, sauté onions and garlic in 1/2 tbsp oil. Mix flax egg together in a small bowl and set aside for at least 10 mins while you prepare the rest of the ingredients.
2. Place all ingredients (except spices and salt) into a large mixing bowl and stir very well. Now, add seasonings and salt to taste.
3. With slightly wet hands, shape dough into patties. Pack dough tightly as this will help it stick together (approx 8 patties)
4. Cooking methods: You can fry the burgers in a bit of oil on a skillet over medium heat for about 5 minutes on each side. If baking in the oven, bake for 25-30 mins (15-17 minutes on each side) at 350°F until golden and crisp.

Ginger Chicken Stir-fry

Ingredients
- 12 oz. boneless, skinless chicken breasts (cut into bite sized pieces)
- 1 tbsp. extra virgin olive oil
- 1 clove garlic (minced)
- 1 tbsp. fresh ginger (chopped)
- 1 medium onion (cut into wedges)
- 1 red bell pepper (cut into strips)
- 1 cup broccoli (cut into bite sized pieces)
- 1/2 cup chicken stock (divided)
- 1 tsp. arrowroot powder
- 1 tbsp. wheat free tamari or Bragg's soy sauce
- 2 cups brown rice (cooked) (GF-sub 3 cups shredded cabbage or Cauliflower Rice)

Preparation:

1. Heat oil in large skillet or wok and add chicken. Cook for approximately 5 minutes. Remove and set aside.
2. Add garlic, ginger, onion, peppers, broccoli and 1/4 cup chicken stock to the skillet. Sauté for 5 minutes.
3. Meanwhile, mix the arrowroot powder into the remaining 1/4 cup chicken stock and tamari sauce.
4. Return chicken to skillet, add tamari mixture and boil. Stir until the sauce thickens.
5. Serve over brown rice, shredded cabbage or Cauliflower Rice.

Asian Salmon

Ingredients

- 12 oz. salmon (cut into 2 fillets)
- 1 cup quinoa (cooked)
- 1 cup bok choy (coarsely chopped)
- 1/2 cup shitake mushrooms (sliced)
- 1 green onion (chopped)
- 1 tbsp. extra virgin olive oil
- 1 tsp. fresh ginger (grated or chopped)
- 1 clove garlic (minced)
- 2 tbsp. wheat free tamari or Bragg's soy sauce
- 2 tsp. sesame oil

Preparation:

1. Preheat oven to 450.
2. Take two 12 x 24 sheets of aluminium foil and fold each sheet over to make a double thick square.
3. Brush a little oil on the centre of each square.
4. Rinse the fish and prepare all of the ingredients.
5. Spread half of the quinoa on the centre of each foil square and then layer the greens, shitake mushrooms, fish and scallions on top.
6. In a small bowl, combine the olive oil, grated ginger, garlic, soy sauce and sesame oil.
7. Pour half of the sauce over each serving. Fold the foil into airtight packets. Bake for 20 minutes.
8. To serve, open the foil packets (being careful of the steam) and transfer to a plate or bowl.

Turkey Tacos

Ingredients

- 1/2 onion (diced)
- 2 celery stalks (diced)
- 2 carrots (peeled and diced)
- 2 tbsp. extra virgin olive oil
- 1 lb. ground turkey
- 2 clove garlic (minced)
- 1/2 cup tomato paste
- 1 tbsp. chilli powder
- 1/2 tsp. cumin
- 1/4 cup cilantro (chopped)

- 6 Gluten Free tortillas (GF-sub Grain Free Wrap or Large Romaine or Butter leaf lettuce leaves)
- 1/2 cup fresh salsa
- 1/2 cup plain 0% Greek yogurt
- 1 1/2 cups salad greens (shredded)
- 1 cup goat mozzarella or Daiya cheese (shredded) (optional)

Preparation:

1. Heat the olive oil in a large skillet and sauté the onion, celery and carrots until soft, about 8-10 minutes.
2. Crumble the ground turkey into the skillet and add the garlic. Cook until turkey is browned.
3. Stir in the tomato paste, chili powder, cumin and 1/2 cup of water.
4. Simmer for about 10-15 minutes. Add cilantro and season with sea salt and pepper to taste.
5. Scoop desired amount of turkey mixture onto each tortilla or lettuce cup and divide the yogurt, greens and cheese (if using) evenly among the tortillas.

Halibut with Carrots and Leeks

Ingredients

- 3 carrots (thinly sliced)
- 2 leeks ((white parts), sliced)
- 4 halibut fillets (1 inch thick; skin removed)
- 4 tbsp. extra virgin olive oil
- 1/2 cup fresh oregano (chopped)

Preparation:

1. Preheat oven to 375°F.
2. Make 4 parchment squares.
3. Place the carrots and leeks in the centre of each square. Place the halibut on top of the vegetables.
4. Season with salt and pepper. Drizzle with the olive oil.
5. Fold the parchment over several times to seal. Place a single layer on a baking sheet. Bake for 25 minutes. Remove from the oven, and transfer each packet to a plate.

Salmon Parcels

Ingredients

- 2 cups green beans (trimmed)
- 3 lemons
- 4 salmon fillets (skin on)
- 1/4 cup pesto
- 1 tbsp. extra virgin olive oil

Preparation:

1. Preheat oven to 400°F.
2. Cut 4 sheets of aluminium foil for each fillet of salmon. Put a handful of beans in the middle of each piece of foil and lay a salmon fillet on top.
3. For each fillet, scoop a spoonful of pesto over the beans, drizzle with olive oil, squeeze half of a lemon over top and season with salt and pepper.
4. Fold up aluminium foil to seal the packets and place on a baking sheet. Cook for 15 minutes. Remove from oven and serve with lemon wedges.

Chicken Dijonaise

Ingredients

- 2 tbsp. extra virgin olive oil
- 2 tbsp. Dijon mustard
- 1 tbsp. fresh rosemary (chopped)
- 1 tbsp. fresh thyme (chopped)
- 1 clove garlic (minced)
- 1/4 tsp. Himalayan sea salt
- 2 boneless, skinless chicken breasts

Preparation:

1. Combine the olive oil, mustard, rosemary, thyme, garlic, salt and a dash of pepper in a small bowl and mix thoroughly.
2. Preheat the oven to 400°F.
3. Place the chicken in a plastic bag along with the mustard marinade and seal. Shake until the chicken is evenly coated and refrigerate for at least 20 minutes.
4. Place in a baking dish and bake in the oven for about 20 minutes or until cooked through and no longer pink inside.

Turkey Burgers

Ingredients

- 1/4 cup green onion (thinly sliced)
- 1/2 cup celery (finely chopped)
- 2 apples (peeled and diced)
- 1 tbsp. extra virgin olive oil

- 1 1/2 lb. ground turkey breast
- Himalayan sea salt and pepper (to taste)
- 1 tsp. Tabasco sauce
- 1 lemon (grated zest and juiced)
- 1 tbsp. fresh dill (chopped)
- 1/4 cup Major Grey chutney
- 1 avocado (sliced)
- 6 Gluten Free whole grain buns (GF-eliminate bun or sub large leaf Romaine or Butter lettuce)

Preparation:
1. Heat the olive oil in a medium skillet on medium high heat. Sauté the onion, celery and apples until soft.
2. In a large mixing bowl, combine the ground turkey with the sautéed ingredients and then mix in remaining ingredients.
3. Form into patties.
4. Place the burgers on a preheated grill and cook for about 6-7 minutes on each side.
5. Place on bun or in lettuce wrap along with sliced avocado.

Chicken and Wild Rice Salad

Ingredients
- *1 cup wild rice (rinsed) (GF-sub Cauliflower Rice)*
- 1 tsp. Himalayan sea salt
- 1 cup cooked chicken
- 1/2 cup celery (chopped)
- 1/2 cup pecans (chopped)

- 2 oranges
- 1/2 cup Balsamic vinaigrette dressing
- 1/4 cup celery leaves

Preparation:
1. In a medium pot, place the salt and rice in 3 cups of water, cover and bring to a boil. *(GF- Make Cauliflower Rice)*
2. Reduce heat and cook slowly until the rice is tender, about 45 minutes.
3. Place the rice or cauliflower rice, chicken, celery and nuts in a large bowl and combine.
4. Slice off both ends of the oranges and using a sharp knife, remove strips of the peel, following the curve of the orange. Then slice between the "lines" to make segments. Cut these segments in half to create bite sized pieces. Add the oranges to the salad.
5. Toss the salad with the vinaigrette and celery leaves and serve.

Turkey Lettuce Wraps

Ingredients
- 1.5 lb. lean ground turkey
- ½ tsp. garlic powder
- 1 tsp. cumin
- 1 tsp. Himalayan sea salt
- 1 tsp. chili powder
- 1 tsp. paprika
- 1/2 tsp. oregano
- 1/2 small onion, minced
- 2 tbsp. bell pepper, minced
- 3/4 cup water

- 4 oz. can tomato sauce
- 8 large lettuce leaves from Romaine or Butter lettuce

Preparation:

1. Brown turkey in a large skillet. When no longer pink add dry seasoning and mix well.
2. Add onion, pepper, water and tomato sauce and cover. Simmer on low for about 20 minutes.
3. Wash and dry the lettuce. Place meat in the centre of leaf and top with tomatoes and salsa.

Sesame Garlic Chicken with Tahini Spinach & Toasted Pecan Quinoa

Ingredients

- 2 boneless, skinless chicken breasts
- 1 clove garlic, minced
- 2 tsp. unsalted sesame seeds, divided
- 3 tbsp. unsalted raw pecans
- ½ cup quinoa (GF-sub Cauliflower Rice)
- 4 cups spinach, washed

Tahini Sauce

- 1 ½ tbsp. sesame tahini
- 1 tsp. rice wine vinegar
- 1 tsp. wheat free tamari or Bragg's soy sauce
- 1/2 tsp. Stevia powder or 1 tsp. Xylitol

Preparation:

1. Ensure that 2 racks are in middle positions in oven. Preheat oven to 375°F.
2. Place chicken on a foil-lined baking pan. With a sharp knife, make 3 slits, a quarter to halfway through each chicken breast. Stuff thin slits with garlic, dividing evenly. Sprinkle 1 tsp. sesame seeds on top of chicken. Place in oven on middle rack and bake for 30 to 35 minutes, until chicken's juices run clear and no pink remains.
3. Meanwhile, on a separate foil-lined baking pan, toast pecans in the same 375 degree F oven for 4 to 6 minutes on top rack.
4. Rinse quinoa thoroughly with water in a fine-mesh strainer until water runs clear. Drain well. Combine quinoa and 1 cup water in a medium-size saucepan. Bring to a boil, then reduce heat to medium-low, cover and cook until grains become translucent, about 15 to 20 minutes. Add toasted pecans to cooked quinoa. *(GF- Make Cauliflower Rice)*
5. Prepare Tahini Sauce: In a small bowl, whisk together tahini, vinegar, soy sauce, 1 tsp. water and Stevia or Xylitol until combined.
6. Divide spinach between 2 plates and top with Tahini Sauce. Sprinkle remaining ½ tsp. sesame seeds on top of spinach. Place chicken breasts and quinoa or cauliflower beside the spinach. Chicken can be kept stored in refrigerator for 4 days.

Rainbow Collard Wraps

Ingredients

- ¼ cup Hummus
- 4 large collard greens
- 2 cups chicken breast thinly sliced or ground turkey
- ½ cup red pepper, thinly sliced
- ½ cup shredded red cabbage
- ½ cup grated beets

- ½ cup grated carrots
- ¼ cup green onions, finely chopped

Preparation:
1. Lay collard greens flat on a cutting board and remove the stems, keeping the leaves connected at the top.
2. Spread 1-2 tbsp. of hummus on each leaf.
3. Top with chicken or turkey. Layer the vegetables on top.
4. Wrap each collard leaf like a burrito, folding the bottom up first, then the sides, then continuing to roll until all the contents are tucked inside.

Lemon Herb Chicken with Zucchini Relish

Ingredients
- 2 tbsp. coconut oil, divided
- 1 lb. chicken, breast, diced
- 1 lime, squeezed
- 1 tbsp. fresh marjoram, chopped, or 1-2 tsp. dried
- ½ tsp. Himalayan sea salt
- ¼ tsp. black pepper
- 1 red onion, diced
- 3 zucchinis, diced
- 1 tbsp. fresh oregano, chopped, or 1-2 tsp. dried
- 1 lemon, squeezed
- Sea salt, to taste; black pepper, to taste

Preparation:

1. Marinate diced chicken in lime juice for 10 minutes.
2. Heat 1 tbsp. coconut oil in a medium skillet to medium heat and cook the chicken with the lime juice. Sprinkle with marjoram and stir occasionally, cooking until no longer pink. Season with salt and pepper. Set aside.
3. Sauté onions in a large skillet with remaining coconut oil over medium heat until soft and translucent. Add zucchini and cook about 8 minutes or until zucchini is soft. Add chopped oregano and lemon juice. Season with salt and pepper. Top chicken with relish.

Coconut Ginger Salmon

Ingredients

- 1/2 onion, diced
- 1 tbsp. coconut oil
- 1 tbsp. ginger root, grated
- ½ tsp. ground fennel
- ½ tsp. cinnamon
- 1 cup coconut milk
- 1 tbsp. lemon juice
- ½ tbsp. lemon zest
- 1/3 lb. wild salmon
- ¼ cup fresh cilantro, chopped, or 1-2 tsp. dried
- Himalayan sea salt, to taste

Preparation:

1. Sauté the onion in the oil until onions are translucent, about 8 minutes. Add the ginger, spices and cook for another 2 minutes.

2. Add the coconut milk, lemon juice and zest and stir to combine. Place the whole fish fillet into the sauce and cook over low heat for about 7-10 minutes or until fish flakes away with a fork at the thickest part.
3. Garnish with chopped cilantro and salt to taste.

Coconut Fried Chicken

Ingredients
- 1 lb. boneless and skinless chicken thighs
- 1 cup coconut milk
- 1 ½ cups coconut flour
- ½ tsp. Himalayan sea salt
- ¼ tsp. black pepper
- 4 tbsp. coconut oil
- 1 cup unsweetened coconut meat

Preparation:
1. In a medium bowl, combine the flour, salt and pepper. In another medium bowl, add the coconut milk. In a third bowl, place the dried coconut meat.
2. Dip each chicken thigh into the coconut milk, then dip into the flour mixture. Cover the chicken completely with the flour. Dip the chicken in the coconut milk again, then dredge in the dried coconut meat. Place the chicken on a plate until you have breaded all the chicken.
3. Heat a non-stick skillet to medium heat with 1-2 tbsp. of coconut oil to start.
4. Cook chicken in the oil over medium heat. Make sure there is plenty of oil and the pan does not get dry. This will prevent burning and also help the chicken to fry. Cook each side about 10 minutes or until chicken is cooked through and browned on the outside.

Saffron Lemon Chicken

Ingredients

- 1 lb. chicken breast, whole
- 1 cup coconut milk
- ½ lemon, squeezed
- ½ tbsp. lemon zest
- ½ tsp. saffron
- ½ tsp. Himalayan sea salt
- ¼ tsp. red pepper
- 2 tsp. fresh parsley, chopped, or 1-2 tsp. dried
- 1/2 cup frozen organic peas

Preparation:

1. Pound the chicken with a meat mallet to tenderize the meat.
2. Pour the coconut milk and lemon juice into a wide saucepan with a lid. Add the saffron, lemon zest and stir gently into the coconut milk.
3. Bring mixture to a low boil, add the whole chicken breasts, reduce the heat to a simmer and cover for 10 minutes, or until the chicken is just cooked through. Add the green peas and cook for one more minute.
4. Salt and pepper to taste and sprinkle the dried or fresh parsley over the chicken to garnish.
5. Serve chicken with saffron-lemon sauce drizzled on top.

Turkey and Quinoa Mix Up

Ingredients
- 2 tbsp. extra virgin olive oil
- 2 cloves garlic, minced
- 1 tsp. Paprika
- 1 tsp. cumin seeds
- 1 tsp. Himalayan sea salt
- ½ tsp. Black pepper
- 1 tsp. cayenne pepper
- 1 onion, minced
- 3 plum tomatoes, diced
- 1 red bell pepper, chopped
- 1 can organic BPA free black beans, rinsed
- 1 can organic BPA free white kidney beans, rinsed
- 1 cup organic non-GMO frozen corn
- 1 lime, juiced
- 1 lb. ground turkey
- *1 cup quinoa (GF-sub cauliflower Rice)*

Preparation:
1. Heat 1 tbsp. olive oil in a saucepan over medium heat. Sauté garlic and paprika, stirring, for about 30 seconds.
2. Add the quinoa and 2 cups of water. Bring to a boil. Reduce heat, cover and let simmer until quinoa is tender and no water remains, about 15 minutes. *(GF-Make Cauliflower Rice)*
3. In a large skillet, heat remaining 1 tbsp. olive oil over medium heat. Sauté the cumin, coriander, salt, pepper and cayenne for a couple of minutes.

4. Add the ground turkey (breaking into small pieces), the onion and pepper and cook until the turkey is no longer pink, about 20 minutes.
5. Add the tomatoes, beans and corn to the skillet and mix well. Cook for another 5 minutes.
6. Add the quinoa or cauliflower ice and lime juice and stir.

Mini Zesty Meatloaves

For the Meatloaf
- 2 lbs. extra lean free range ground beef (or lean ground turkey)
- 2 eggs, beaten
- 2 carrots, grated
- 1 bell pepper, finely chopped
- 1 onion, chopped
- 2 cloves garlic, minced
- 1 tbsp. coconut oil
- 1 tsp. cumin
- 1 tsp. chili powder
- ½ tsp. Himalayan sea salt
- ½ tsp. Black pepper

For the Sauce
- 7 oz. tomato paste
- ½ cup water
- 1 tbsp. fresh cilantro leaves
- ½ tsp. chili powder
- Himalayan sea salt and black pepper to taste
- ¼ cup chopped red bell pepper

Preparation:

1. Preheat the oven to 375°F. Line 2 mini loaf pans or 1 large loaf pan with parchment paper.
2. In a small sauce pan over medium heat, combine the tomato paste, water, bell pepper, cilantro, chili powder and a dash of salt and pepper.
3. Simmer for 5-10 minutes stirring occasionally. Set aside.
4. Melt the coconut oil in a medium skillet. Sauté the onion until translucent and browned.
5. In a large mixing bowl combine the cooked onion, garlic, cumin, chili powder, salt, pepper, carrots, bell pepper and mix well.
6. Add the eggs and ground meat- mix well to combine.
7. Divide the mixture into the 2 loaf pans.
8. Spoon ¼ cup of the sauce onto each of the loaves and reserve the remaining sauce for dipping after the loaves are baked.
9. Bake uncovered for approximately 45 minutes (65 min for a larger single loaf).

Chicken with Asparagus and Almond Pesto

Ingredients

- 1 lb. asparagus, trimmed
- 2 cups cherry tomatoes
- 3 tbsp. extra virgin olive oil
- ½ cup sliced almonds
- ¼ cup fresh basil leaves, or 1 tbsp. dried
- Himalayan sea salt and black pepper to taste
- 4 boneless, skinless chicken breasts

Preparation:

1. Preheat the oven to 425°F.
2. Arrange the asparagus on half of a rimmed baking sheet and the tomatoes on the other half. Drizzle with olive oil, season with sea salt and pepper- toss to coat. Roast for about 20 minutes or until the asparagus is bright green and the tomatoes have collapsed. Let cool and remove the tips from the roasted asparagus and set aside.
3. Reserve 1 tbsp. of the almonds and place the rest in a food processor. Roughly chop the asparagus bottoms and place these in the food processor as well along with the basil and 3 tbsp. olive oil. Pulse until a paste forms. Season with salt and pepper.
4. Heat grill. Spread a spoonful of the pesto on top of each chicken breast. Grill until no longer pink inside and juice runs clear.
5. Mix the asparagus tops and tomatoes. Evenly distribute among plates and serve with the grilled chicken breasts. You may wish to spread any leftover pesto over the chicken as well.

Fish N' Shrooms

Ingredients

- 1 tbsp. extra virgin olive oil
- 1 lb. cod or other white fish
- 1 cup fresh mushroom, sliced
- 2 cloves garlic, minced
- 2 green onions, chopped
- ½ lemon, wedged
- Himalayan Sea Salt and Black Pepper

Preparation:

1. Heat the olive oil in a skillet and cook the fish. Season with salt and pepper on both sides and set aside.
2. Add the mushrooms and garlic to the pan and cook until brown. Season to taste with S & P.
3. Add the fish back to the skillet with the scallions and cook for an additional 2 min.
4. Serve with lemon wedges and squeeze over fish.

Crock Pot Chicken and Veggie Soup

Ingredients

- 1.5 litres chicken broth
- 1 cup bell peppers, diced
- 2 carrots, grated
- 1 medium zucchini, chopped
- 1 medium onion, chopped
- 2 garlic cloves, minced
- 1 cup broccoli, cut into small florets
- 1 cup cauliflower, cut into small florets
- 1 cup crimini mushrooms, chopped
- 1 tsp. cumin
- 1 tsp. Himalayan sea salt
- ½ tsp. Black pepper
- 2 tsp. parsley
- 2 cups leftover chicken breast, chopped
- ½ cup quinoa, rinsed (optional)(GF- Leave out)

Preparation:

1. Add all ingredients to crock pot and cook on low for 8 hours or on high for 4 hours.

Black Bean and Sweet Potato Chili

Ingredients

- 2 medium sized sweet potatoes
- 2 tbsp. extra virgin olive oil
- 1 medium sized onion, chopped
- 3 cloves garlic, minced
- 1 red bell pepper, diced
- 2 cans organic BPA free black beans
- 28 oz. can organic BPA diced tomatoes
- 4 oz. can chopped green chilies
- 2 tsp. cumin
- ½ tsp. oregano
- Himalayan sea salt and Black pepper to taste
- Fresh cilantro (to garnish)

Preparation:

1. Bake sweet potatoes at 350°F degrees until slightly firm, but not soft. When cool, peel and dice into ¾ inch cubes. Set aside.
2. Heat oil in soup pot or Dutch oven. Add garlic and onion and sauté over medium heat until golden brown.
3. Add remaining ingredients and heat. Cover and simmer for 15 minutes.
4. Add diced sweet potatoes and continue to simmer until vegetables are tender, 10-15 minutes. Add salt to taste.

5. Taste improves if allowed to stand for 1-2 hours before serving. Reheat and serve with chopped cilantro for garnish.

Basic Grilled Chicken

Ingredients
- 4-6 boneless, skinless chicken breasts
- 1 lemon, juiced (for a variation 2 tbsp. balsamic vinegar can be substituted)
- 1 tsp. dried oregano, parsley, rosemary or other herbs
- ½ tsp. Himalayan sea salt
- ½ tsp. Black pepper
- 2 tbsp. coconut oil (for grill method only)
- 2 tbsp. extra virgin olive oil

Preparation:
1. Butterfly chicken breasts (Cut the chicken breast in half through the thickest part of the breast).
2. Combine lemon juice or balsamic vinegar and herbs in a large bowl.
3. Add chicken breasts and turn evenly to coat. Allow to marinate for at least 5 minutes.
4. Heat a grill pan or grill to medium heat and brush the grill with coconut oil. Cook chicken for 4 to 5 minutes per side. Once complete brush the cooked chicken with olive oil and allow to rest for 5 minutes.
5. Alternatively pre-heat oven to 350°F. Line a baking sheet with parchment paper. Bake chicken breasts for 45 minutes or until there is no pink in the centre. Once complete, brush the cooked chicken with olive oil and allow to rest for 5 minutes.

Sides and Salads

Cauliflower Celery Root Mash

Ingredients

- 1 medium celery root (about 16 ounces), peeled and cut into 1/2-inch cubes
- 1 small head or half a large head of cauliflower (about 16 ounces), cut into small florets
- ½ tsp. Himalayan Sea salt
- 3 tbsp. organic grass fed butter (or coconut oil)

Preparation:

1. Trim and skin celery root and cut into 1 inch cubes.
2. Cut cauliflower into small florets.
3. Steam the celery root and cauliflower florets until fork tender (approx. 15 minutes)
4. Transfer vegetables to the bowl of a food processor, add butter or coconut oil and salt and process until smooth (you may need to add 1 or 2 Tablespoons of the steaming liquid to loosen the puree to the right consistency). Season with additional salt and pepper to taste.

Cauliflower Rice

Ingredients

- 1 head cauliflower
- 1 tablespoon extra-virgin olive oil
- 1 medium onion, diced
- Coarse salt and coarsely-ground black pepper to taste
- Spices, herbs, and/or vegetables of your choice

Preparation:
1. Wash and trim cauliflower.
2. Grate cauliflower with cheese grater to rice like consistency. This can also be done in a food processor.
3. Add olive oil to sauté pan along with onion. Sauté until softened.
4. If adding other vegetables, do so at this point and sauté.
5. Add cauliflower rice and sauté for 4-5 min. so that it is still slightly crunchy.

Steamed Veggies and Greens

Ingredients
- 1 bunch kale, washed and chopped, rib removed
- 1 bunch chard, washed and chopped, rib removed
- 1 zucchini chopped
- 1 cup shitake or brown mushrooms, chopped
- 1 tsp. freshly grated ginger
- 2 cloves garlic minced
- 2 tbsp. coconut oil

Preparation:
1. Sautee all ingredients together.

Italian Veggies with Artichoke Hearts

Ingredients
- 1 tbsp. coconut oil
- ½ red onion, diced

- 1 zucchini, sliced
- 1 cup green beans, cut into 2 inch pieces
- 4 cups spinach leaves
- 1 cup artichoke hearts, halved
- ½ lemon, squeezed
- Himalayan sea salt, to taste
- ¼ tsp. black pepper
- 1 tsp. dried basil
- 1 tsp. dried oregano

Preparation:
1. Heat the coconut oil in a sauté pan over medium heat.
2. Cook the onions for about 8 minutes on medium heat or until cooked through.
3. Add the green beans and zucchini and sauté about 5-8 minutes or until almost cooked.
4. Add the spinach and sauté another 5-8 minutes until cooked through.
5. Add the lemon juice, artichoke hearts, salt, pepper and herbs. Heat through another 5 minutes.

Twisted Asparagus

Ingredients
- 2 cloves garlic (minced)
- 1 tbsp. raw honey
- 1 tsp. wheat free tamari or Bragg's soy sauce
- 1 tbsp. extra virgin olive oil
- 1 tsp. sesame oil

- 1 lb. asparagus
- 1 tsp. sesame seeds

Preparation:

1. Mix garlic, honey, tamari and oil in a small bowl.
2. Heat skillet over medium heat and pour mixture into pan.
3. Add asparagus and cook until tender crisp.
4. Sprinkle with sesame seeds and serve.

Steamed Broccoli with Herbs

Ingredients

- 1 head broccoli, chopped into florets
- 2 tbsp. coconut oil or extra virgin olive oil
- ½ tsp. Himalayan sea salt
- 1 tsp. dried chives
- 1 tbsp. fresh parsley

Preparation:

1. Steam or boil the broccoli florets until tender but still bright green, about 8-10 minutes. Transfer broccoli to a serving dish.
2. Combine the coconut oil or olive oil, salt and herbs- drizzle over the broccoli.

Mashed Cauliflower

Ingredients

- 1 head cauliflower
- ½ tsp. Himalayan sea salt
- ¼ tsp. black pepper
- 2 tbsp. coconut oil

Preparation:

1. Steam the cauliflower in a large pot for about 10-15 minutes or just until soft. Drain the cauliflower.
2. Add the steamed cauliflower, salt and butter or oil to a food processor. Process until smooth.

Lemony Green Beans

Ingredients

- 1 tbsp. coconut oil
- ½ tbsp. ginger root, freshly grated, or 1/2 tsp. dried
- 2 cloves garlic, minced
- 1 lb. green beans, stems removed
- 1 lemon, squeezed
- 1 tsp. lemon zest
- 1 tsp. dried basil
- 2 tbsp. water
- Himalayan sea salt, to taste

Preparation:

1. In a cast iron skillet or non-stick pan, heat the coconut oil to medium-high heat. Add ginger and garlic and sauté for 1 minute.
2. Add the green beans, lemon juice, zest and 2 tbsp. of water. Sauté/steam over medium heat for 10 minutes, stirring occasionally.
3. Add the salt and basil and continue cooking the beans until they are soft but not overcooked. Add a bit more water or oil if needed.

Mashed Cauliflower

Ingredients

- 1 large head cauliflower
- 5 large cloves garlic, minced
- ½ tsp. Himalayan sea salt
- 2 tablespoons grass-fed butter or coconut oil
- ¼ teaspoon freshly ground nutmeg
- Freshly ground black pepper to taste

Preparation:

1. Steam the cauliflower and garlic for 15 minutes or until completely soft.
2. Add all ingredients to a food processor and blend until smooth (alternatively use a potato masher and mash until smooth).

Baked Yams

Ingredients

- 2-4 medium sized yams, skinned and cut into ½ inch medallions
- 1-2 tbsp. coconut oil
- ½ tsp. Himalayan sea salt

Preparation:

1. Pre-heat oven to 350°F.
2. Place yams into oven safe cook ware (such as corning ware).
3. Coat with coconut oil and sea salt
4. Bake covered for 40 minutes or until fork tender. Bake uncovered for 5-10 minutes or until edges are slightly browned.

Yam Fries

Ingredients

- 2-4 medium sized yams
- 2 tbsp. extra virgin olive oil
- 1 tsp. Himalayan sea salt

Preparation:

1. Pre-heat oven to 375°F.
2. Line a baking pan with parchment paper.
3. Cut yams into French fry lengths.
4. Coat sliced yams with olive oil and sprinkle with sea salt.
5. Bake yams uncovered for 45 minutes or until tender and crisp.

Chickpea Salad

Ingredients

- 1 can chickpeas, rinsed
- 1 zucchini, chopped
- 1 tomato, chopped
- 1 bunch kale, chopped
- 2 tbsp. apple cider vinegar
- Himalayan sea salt to taste
- 2 tbsp. nutritional yeast
- 1 tbsp. coconut oil

Preparation:

1. Sautee zucchini, tomatoes and kale in 1 tbsp. coconut oil until soft- let cool.
2. In a bowl add chickpeas, cooled veggie mixture, vinegar, nutritional yeast and salt.

5 Spice Chicken and Orange Salad

Ingredients

- 6 tbsp. extra virgin olive oil (divided)
- 1 tsp. 5 spice powder
- 1 tsp. Himalayan sea salt (divided)
- 1/2 tsp. black pepper
- 1 lb. boneless, skinless chicken breasts
- 3 oranges
- 1 red bell pepper
- 1/2 cup red onion (thinly sliced)

- 1 tbsp. cider vinegar
- 1 tbsp. Dijon mustard
- 8 cups mixed wild greens

Preparation:
1. Preheat oven to 450°F.
2. Combine 1 tsp. oil, five-spice powder, 1/2 tsp. salt and 1/2 tsp. pepper in a small bowl. Rub the mixture into both sides of the chicken breasts.
3. Heat 1 tsp. oil in a large ovenproof non-stick skillet over medium-high heat. Add chicken breasts; cook until browned on one side, 3 to 5 minutes. Turn them over and transfer the pan to the oven. Roast until the chicken is just cooked through, 6 to 8 minutes. Set chicken aside.
4. Meanwhile, peel and segment two of the oranges, collecting segments and any juice in a large bowl. Add the greens, bell pepper and onion to the bowl. Zest and juice the remaining orange and place in a small bowl.
5. Whisk in vinegar, mustard, the remaining 4 tsp. oil, remaining 1/2 tsp. salt and freshly ground pepper to taste.
6. Pour the dressing over the salad; toss to combine. Slice the chicken and serve on the salad.

Curried Chicken Quinoa Salad

Ingredients
- 2 1/2 cups chicken stock
- 2 cups boneless, skinless chicken breast (thinly sliced)
- 4 tsp. curry powder (divided)
- *2 cups quinoa, cooked (GF-sub Cauliflower Rice)*
- 1 cup red bell pepper (diced)

- 1 can chickpeas (rinsed and drained)
- 1/2 cup green onion (chopped)
- 1/2 cup cilantro (chopped)
- 1/4 cup dried cranberries
- 1 tbsp. Dijon mustard
- 6 drops hot sauce
- 4 cups wild greens salad
- 2 tomatoes (sliced)

Preparation:
1. In a medium pan, bring the chicken stock to a boil over medium heat.
2. Poach chicken pieces in the stock until cooked through, about 3-5 minutes. Remove to a plate. Toss chicken with 1 1/2 teaspoons curry powder and set aside.
3. Return the broth to a boil, add the quinoa and stir. Cover and simmer 15 minutes. (GF-Make Cauliflower Rice)
4. Place quinoa or Cauliflower Rice in a mixing bowl and fluff. Stir in the bell pepper, chickpeas, green onion, cilantro and cranberries.
5. Add the Dijon, remaining curry powder and hot sauce and stir until combined.
6. Arrange salad greens and tomato slices on 4 plates and spoon quinoa or cauliflower rice salad over top.

Spinach Salad

Ingredients
- 4 cups spinach, washed
- 1/2 cup strawberries (sliced)
- 1/4 cup pecans

- 1/4 cup goat feta (crumbled)
- 1/4 cup balsamic vinaigrette

Preparation:
1. Toss first four ingredients together.
2. Mix salad dressing to coat and serve

Wild Greens Salad

Ingredients
- ½ cup carrot (grated)
- ½ cup red pepper (chopped)
- 1 cup cucumber (diced)
- 10 cherry tomatoes (halved)
- 1/4 cup cranberry trail mix
- 1tbsp. balsamic vinaigrette dressing
- 4 cups mixed wild greens

Preparation:
1. Place all ingredients in a large bowl.
2. Drizzle balsamic dressing over salad

Orange Spinach Salad

Ingredients
- 6 cups spinach, washed
- 1/2 cup mandarin oranges, in water

- 1/4 cup pecans (roughly chopped)
- 1/4 cup balsamic vinaigrette

Preparation:

1. Combine all ingredients and toss

Red Quinoa and Black Bean Salad

For the salad:

- *1 cup uncooked Red quinoa (GF-sub Cauliflower Rice or 2 cups shredded cabbage)*
- 1 can black beans, drained and rinsed
- 1 red pepper, chopped
- 1/4 cup fresh Cilantro, finely chopped
- 2 green onions, chopped
- 1 cup fresh or frozen Non-GMO Organic corn (optional)
- 1 small avocado, chopped into 1 inch pieces

For the dressing:

- 4-5 tbsp. of fresh lime juice (juice from 2 small limes)
- 1/2 tsp. Himalayan sea salt
- 1/2 tsp. freshly ground black pepper
- 1 garlic clove, minced
- 1/4 cup fresh Cilantro, finely chopped
- 1/4 cup extra virgin olive oil
- 1/2 tsp. ground cumin, or more to taste

Preparation:

1. Cook 1 cup red quinoa with 2 cups water. Bring to a boil. Cover and simmer 15minutes. *(GF- Make Cauliflower Rice).*
2. While quinoa is cooking, prepare the chopped vegetables and whisk together the dressing.
3. Allow quinoa to cool after cooking for about 5 minutes. Fluff with a fork. Add the beans and vegetables and toss well.
4. Drizzle dressing over salad. Toss well with salt and pepper to taste. Bring salad to room temperature before serving. Keep fresh in a sealed container for 1-2 days. Makes about 5 cups.

Protein Power Bowl

Ingredients

- 1 cup uncooked green lentils or 1 can organic lentils, rinsed
- *1 cup brown rice, cooked (GF-leave out or sub Cauliflower Rice)*
- 1/2 tbsp. extra virgin olive oil
- 1/2 red onion, chopped
- 3-4 garlic cloves, minced
- 1 red bell pepper, chopped
- 1 large tomato, chopped
- 3 cups spinach or kale, roughly chopped
- 1/2 cup fresh parsley, minced
- 1 cup Tahini-Lemon Dressing (recipe below)
- Himalayan sea salt & black pepper, to taste
- Lemon Wedges & lemon zest, to garnish

Tahini dressing

- 3 garlic cloves
- 1/2 cup fresh lemon juice (about 2 lemons)
- 1/4 cup Nutritional yeast
- 2 tbsp. extra virgin olive oil
- 1 tsp. Himalayan sea salt + freshly ground black pepper, or to taste
- 3 tbsp water, or as needed
- ¼ cup tahini

Tahini Dressing Directions

1. In a food processor, add all ingredients and process until smooth. Makes just under 1 cup.

Preparation:

1. Cook lentils with 2 cups water. Bring to a boil and simmer uncovered for 20-30 minutes. Set aside to cool.
2. Prepare the tahini dressing in food processor.
3. In a large skillet over low-medium heat, add olive oil and sauté the chopped onion and minced garlic for a few minutes, being careful not to burn. Add in the chopped red pepper and tomato and sauté for another 7-8 minutes.
4. Stir in the chopped kale or spinach and sauté for another few minutes, just until tender. Stir in the full batch of tahini dressing, the cooked & drained grains or cauliflower rice and lentils. Simmer on low for another few minutes.
5. Remove from heat and stir in the minced parsley.
6. Season with salt and pepper to taste and garnish with lemon wedges and zest. Makes 6 cups.

Weekend Kale Salad

Ingredients

- 1/2 large head of kale (about 4-6 cups)
- ½ cup finely chopped red onion
- 1/2 red bell pepper
- 1/2 cup chopped carrot
- 1 English cucumber, chopped
- 1 avocado, chopped
- 1 cup cherry tomato, chopped
- 1/2 cup mixed raisins and Goji berries
- 1/4 cup hemp seed
- 1/3 cup chopped walnuts
- Dressing: 1 cup of Tahini-Lemon Dressing (See Recipe)

Tahini dressing

- 3 garlic cloves
- 1/2 cup fresh lemon juice (about 2 lemons)
- 1/4 cup Nutritional yeast
- 2 tbsp. extra virgin olive oil
- 1 tsp. Himalayan sea salt and freshly ground black pepper, or to taste
- 3 tbsp. water or as needed
- ¼ cup tahini

Tahini Dressing Directions

1. In a food processor, add all ingredients and process until smooth. Makes just under 1 cup.

Preparation:

1. Chop vegetables and mix in a large mixing bowl. Reserve hemp seed and walnuts for sprinkling on top.
2. Tear the leaves off the kale and rip into bite-sized pieces. Wash and dry kale leaves.
3. Mix the vegetables, kale leaves and 1 cup of dressing in large bowl until thoroughly combined.
4. Place in fridge to 'marinate' for 10-15 minutes. Serves 4. Keeps in fridge in a sealed container for 1 day.

Green Salad with Pumpkin Seeds

Ingredients

- 4 cups mixed salad greens
- 2 stalks celery, diced finely
- 1 cucumber, peeled and diced
- 1 cup sunflower sprouts, cut into 1 inch pieces
- 1 avocado, diced
- 1 cup raw pumpkin seeds
- 2 tbsp. apple cider vinegar or lemon juice
- 1/3 cup extra virgin olive oil
- Himalayan sea salt, to taste
- Black pepper to taste
- 1 tsp. dried thyme
- 1 tsp. Dijon mustard

Preparation:

1. Combine the salad greens, cucumber, celery, avocado and sprouts together in a salad bowl. Sprinkle the pumpkin seeds on top.

2. Mix the olive oil, apple cider vinegar, mustard, salt, pepper and thyme together in a small bowl.
3. Drizzle over salad

Wild Green Salad

Ingredients
- 1 carrot, grated
- 1 red pepper, chopped
- ½ cup cucumber, diced
- 10 cherry tomatoes, halved
- 2 tbsp. dried organic cranberries
- 4 cups organic wild greens salad mixture
- 2 tbsp. balsamic vinaigrette

Preparation:
1. Combine all ingredients and top with balsamic vinaigrette

Curry Quinoa Salad

Ingredients
- 2 ½ cups chicken stock *(GF- If subbing Cauliflower Rice reduce chicken stock to 1 cup)*
- 2 cups boneless, skinless chicken breasts, thinly sliced
- 4 tsp. curry powder
- 1 cup red bell pepper, diced
- 1 can organic BPA free chickpeas, rinsed
- ½ cup green onion, chopped

- ½ cup fresh cilantro
- ¼ cup dried organic cranberries
- 2 tbsp. Dijon mustard
- 1 tsp. hot sauce
- 2 cups salad greens
- 3 tomatoes, sliced
- *1 cup quinoa (GF-sub Cauliflower Rice- reduce chicken stock to 1 cup)*

Preparation:

1. In a medium pan, bring the chicken stock to a boil over medium heat.
2. Poach chicken pieces in the stock until cooked through, about 3-5 minutes. Set aside. Toss chicken with 1 ½ teaspoons curry powder and set aside.
3. Return the broth to a boil, add the quinoa and stir. Remove pan from heat, cover and let sit for about 5 minutes. *(GF-Make Cauliflower Rice)*
4. Place quinoa or Cauliflower Rice in a mixing bowl and fluff. Stir in the bell pepper, chickpeas, green onion, cilantro and cranberries.
5. Add the Dijon, remaining curry powder and hot sauce. Stir until combined.
6. Arrange salad greens and tomato slices on 4 plates and spoon quinoa or Cauliflower Rice salad over top.

How to Cook Quinoa

Ingredients

- 1 cup quinoa (any variety—white or golden, red, or black)
- 1 tbsp. extra virgin olive oil (optional)
- 2 cups liquid, such as broth or water
- ¼ tsp. Himalayan sea salt (optional)

Preparation:

1. **Rinse the quinoa.** Place the quinoa in a fine-mesh strainer and rinse thoroughly with cool water. Rub and swish the quinoa with your hand while rinsing and rinse for at least 2 minutes under the running water. Drain.

(Rinsing removes quinoa's natural coating, called *saponin*, which can make it taste bitter or soapy)

2. **Dry and toast quinoa in saucepan.** Heat a drizzle of olive oil in the saucepan over medium-high heat and add the drained quinoa. Cook, stirring, for about 1 minute, letting the water evaporate.
3. **Add liquid and bring to a boil. Add in sea salt, if using.**
4. **Lower heat and cook covered for 15 minutes**
5. **Let stand covered for 5 minutes.**
6. After 5 minutes, remove the lid. Fluff the quinoa gently with a fork and serve. (You should see tiny spirals (the germ) separating from and curling around the quinoa seeds.)

Baking and Sneaky Treats

Seed Flatbread

Ingredients

- 1 ½ cups raw pumpkin seeds, ground into flour
- 1 ½ cups sunflower seeds, ground into flour
- 1 tsp. Himalayan sea salt
- 2 tbsp. ground flax meal
- 6 tbsp. boiling water
- 2 tsp. extra virgin olive oil

- 1-2 pinches green leaf stevia powder (optional)
- 1/2 tsp. garlic powder or 1 garlic clove, minced
- 1 tsp. dried basil
- 1 tsp. dried parsley

Preparation:
1. Preheat oven to 350° F. Grind the seeds before measuring out 1 cup flour of each to total 2 cups of flour.
2. Combine the flax seed meal and hot water and let sit for 5 minutes.
3. Combine all ingredients together in a mixing bowl. Knead the dough until everything is mixed. The dough will be very stiff. Add more pumpkin or sunflower seed flour if dough seems too wet and a little more olive oil if dough seems too dry.
4. Grease a pizza sheet and sprinkle it with coarsely ground pumpkin seeds. Pat the dough into a ball shape and place it in the middle of the cookie sheet. Beginning in the center and moving outwards, squish the dough flat with your hands. Use a rolling pin or even a drinking glass to roll out the dough.
5. Bake for 20 minutes until browned (or long longer if not cooked through). Remove from heat and enjoy as a pizza or as a flat bread with veggies.

Paleo Almond Snack Muffins

Ingredients
- 1 cup almond butter
- 1 cup sliced almonds
- 1 cup pure coconut milk
- 2 cups unsweetened shredded coconut
- 3 eggs

- 1/4 tsp. vanilla extract (optional)
- 2 Tbsp. coconut sap or raw honey (optional)
- 12 paper muffin liners

Preparation:

1. Preheat oven to 400°F.
2. Line a muffin tin with paper liners.
3. Combine all ingredients and pour into muffin tin.
4. Bake for 15 minutes.

Paleo Pumpkin Snack Muffins

Ingredients

- 1½ cups almond flour
- ¾ cup canned pumpkin (or cook and puree pumpkin yourself)
- 3 large eggs
- 1 tsp. baking powder
- 1 tsp. baking soda
- ½ tsp. ground cinnamon
- 1½ tsp. pumpkin pie spice
- 1/8 tsp. sea salt
- ¼ cup raw honey (optional)
- 2 tsp. almond butter
- 1 tbsp. sliced almonds

Preparation:

1. Preheat oven to 350°F.
2. Coat muffin tins with coconut oil (or use paper muffin cups and add 1/2 tsp. melted coconut oil to batter).
3. Mix all ingredients and pour evenly into tins.
4. Bake for 25 minutes on the middle rack.
5. Sprinkle almonds on top immediately after taking them out of the oven.

Paleo Blueberry Snack Muffins

Ingredients

- ½ cup coconut flour, sifted
- ½ tsp. baking soda
- ½ tsp. Himalayan sea salt
- ¼ tsp. nutmeg
- ½ tsp. cinnamon
- 6 eggs
- 1/3 cup raw honey
- ¼ cup coconut oil, melted
- 1 tbsp. vanilla extract
- 1 cup fresh blueberries
- Zest of 1 lemon

Preparation:

1. In a small bowl, combine coconut flour, baking soda, salt, nutmeg and cinnamon.
2. In a large bowl, combine eggs, honey, oil and vanilla. Blend well with whisk.
3. Mix dry ingredients into wet, blending with a whisk.

4. Fold in blueberries and lemon zest with a spatula.
5. Pour batter evenly into a 12 cup muffin tin (greased with coconut oil or if using paper liners).
6. Bake at 350°F for 15 to 20 minutes.

Almond Butter Cups

Ingredients
- 1/3 cup coconut oil
- 1/3 cup raw carob powder
- 1/3 cup almond butter

Preparation:
1. Line a cookie sheet with 12 mini cupcake wrappers.
2. Mix all ingredients in a medium mixing bowl. Combine until smooth.
3. Place 1 tsp. of mixture into each cupcake wrapper. Freeze.
4. Keep in freezer in freezer proof bag and enjoy one as a treat.

Grain Free Wrap

Ingredients
- 3 tbsp. ground flaxseed
- 1/4 tsp. baking powder (aluminum free)
- Pinch of Himalayan sea salt
- 1 tbsp. melted coconut oil
- 3 tbsp. water
- 1 large egg or you can use 3 tbsp. boxed egg whites

Preparation:

1. Mix all the dry ingredients together and set aside.
2. Mix all the wet ingredients together and pour into the dry ingredients.
3. Melt a drop of coconut oil in a frying pan, until just melted. Remove pan from heat. Pour in the batter and very gently work into the shape of a pancake with even distribution.
4. Once done, place pan back on the stove and cook over low heat until you see the batter start to rise and get crisp along the edges. Gently turn and cook until done.
5. You can make a larger batch and store in the fridge for a couple of days.

Coconut Macaroons

Ingredients

- 4 large egg whites
- 1 ½ cups unsweetened rough coconut
- 1 tbsp. xylitol
- ½ tsp. vanilla extract

Preparation:

1. Add the egg whites and vanilla to a medium sized mixing bowl.
2. Beat the egg whites until they become firm and peak.
3. Once the eggs are stiff, add the coconut and stevia- fold in very gently.
4. Line a cookie sheet with parchment paper and, with a spoon, drop the mixture onto the cookie sheet.
5. Bake at 350°F degrees for 15 minutes.
6. Remove from pan and place on rack to cool.

No Bake Energy Bites

Ingredients

- 1 cup dry oatmeal
- 2/3 cup coconut flakes
- ½ cup organic peanut butter
- ½ cup ground flax seeds
- ½ cup dairy free chocolate chips
- 1/3 cup raw honey
- 1 tbsp. Chia seeds
- 1 tsp. vanilla extract

Preparation:

1. Mix all ingredients together and let sit in fridge for 30 minutes.
2. Roll into small balls about 1 inch in size.
3. Store in air tight container in fridge.
4. Enjoy one as a treat.

Dips, Dressings and Snacks

Hummus

Ingredients

- 2 cloves of garlic
- 1 tbsp. extra virgin olive oil
- 1 can chickpeas
- 4 tbsp. sesame tahini

- 3 tbsp. water
- 1 tsp. Himalayan sea salt
- ¼ cup lemon juice
- ½ tsp. black pepper
- 2 tbsp. chopped fresh parsley (optional)
- ½ tsp. cumin

Preparation:

1. Place all ingredients into a food processor and blend thoroughly.
2. Put in airtight container in the fridge for up to 5 days.

Skinny Guacamole

Ingredients

- 1 large zucchini, cut into 1/2-inch cubes
- 1 large ripe avocado, cubed
- ¼ cup coarsely chopped fresh cilantro
- ¼ cup finely chopped onion
- 2 cloves garlic, minced
- 2 tbsp. lime juice
- ½ tsp. hot sauce, such as Tabasco, or more to taste
- ¼ tsp. Himalayan Sea Salt

Preparation:

1. Place zucchini in a microwave-safe glass dish. Cover with a damp paper towel and microwave on high until tender- 4 to 5 minutes. Drain in a sieve, pressing lightly on the zucchini to extract any liquid. Alternatively steam zucchini until tender, approx. 10 minutes.

2. Transfer the zucchini to a large bowl; add avocado, cilantro, onion, garlic, lime juice, hot sauce and sea salt. Coarsely mash until combined.

(Serve with raw veggies, coconut flour tortillas or Mary's gluten free crackers)

Tahini Salad Dressing

Ingredients
- 1 cup chopped celery stalks with leaves
- ¼ cup chopped green bell pepper
- ½ of a medium onion chopped
- 2 garlic cloves, chopped
- ½ cup Braggs Liquid Aminos or Wheat free Tamari
- ¾ cup tahini
- ½ cup lemon juice
- ¾ cup extra virgin olive oil

Preparation:
1. Put everything into a food processor and mix until creamy. Must be refrigerated.

Italian Dressing

Ingredients
- ¼ cup olive oil
- ¼ cup lemon juice
- ¼ cup lime juice
- ¼ cup unsweetened apple juice

- ¼ tsp. oregano
- ½ tsp. dry mustard
- ½ tsp. onion powder
- ½ tsp. paprika
- 1/8 tsp. thyme
- 1/8 tsp. rosemary

Preparation:

1. Place all ingredients into a food processor. Blend until smooth or mix thoroughly in a jar with a lid- can be refrigerated for up to 10 days.

Basic Balsamic Vinaigrette

Ingredients

- ¼ cup balsamic vinegar
- 1 tbsp. chopped garlic
- ½ tsp. salt
- ½ tsp. black pepper freshly ground
- ¾ cup extra-virgin olive oil

Preparation:

1. Place all ingredients into a food processor. Blend until smooth or mix thoroughly in a jar with a lid- can be refrigerated for up to 10 days.

Balsamic Vinaigrette

Ingredients

- 1/3 cup extra virgin olive oil
- 2 tbsp. balsamic vinegar
- ½ tbsp. red wine vinegar
- 1 clove garlic minced or pressed
- ½ tsp. ground mustard
- 1 tbsp. lemon juice

Preparation:

1. Place all ingredients into a food processor. Blend until smooth or mix thoroughly in a jar with a lid-can be refrigerated for up to 10 days.

Skinny Balsamic Vinaigrette

Ingredients

- ½ cup Balsamic Vinegar
- ¼ cup water
- 3 tbsp. extra virgin olive oil
- 1 tbsp. Dijon mustard
- 1 tbsp. garlic, minced
- 1 tsp. raw honey
- Himalayan sea salt & pepper to taste

Preparation:

1. Place all ingredients into a food processor. Blend until smooth or mix thoroughly in a jar with a lid- can be refrigerated for up to 10 days.

Kale Chips

Ingredients

- 1 bunch kale
- 1 tablespoon olive oil
- 1 teaspoon seasoned salt
- (Optional –add ¼ cup nutritional yeast)

Preparation:

1. Preheat an oven to 350°F. Line a non-insulated cookie sheet with parchment paper.
2. With a knife or kitchen shears carefully remove the leaves from the thick stems and tear into bite size pieces. Wash and thoroughly dry kale with a salad spinner. Drizzle kale with olive oil and sprinkle with seasoning salt and nutritional yeast (if using).
3. Bake until the edges are brown but are not burnt- 10 to 15 minutes.

Roasted Chickpea Snack

Ingredients

- 2 tbsp. extra virgin olive oil
- 1 tbsp. ground cumin
- 1 tsp. garlic powder
- 1/2 tsp. chili powder
- Himalayan sea salt and black pepper to taste

- ½ tsp. crushed red pepper
- 1 (15 ounce) can chickpeas, rinsed

Preparation:
1. Preheat an oven to 350°F.
2. Whisk the oil, cumin, garlic powder, chili powder, sea salt, black pepper and red pepper together in a small bowl. Add the chickpeas and toss to coat. Spread into a single layer on a baking sheet.
3. Roast in preheated oven, stirring occasionally, until nicely browned and slightly crispy, about 45 minutes.

Recipe References:

www.eatcleanmenus.com

www.drcobi.com

www.ohsheglows.com

www.nourishingmeals.com

www.heartofcooking.com

www.eatcleandiet.com

www.21daysugardetox.com

Appendix

Recommended Supplements

The following supplements are recommended in each chapter and are available from Dr Cobi's online store on www.drcobi.com or http://store.drcobi.com/

Liver Toxicity:
- Cellular Detox
- DL Detox Pack
- Liver Formula RX
- LVDTX
- LCH
- TAPS
- Fiber Formula
- Medibulk
- Metafiber
- Mediclear, Mediclear Plus, Chocolate Mediclear SGS
- Metabolic Cleanse
- Calcium D Glucarate

Stress and the Adrenals:
- Adrenomend
- Cortrex
- Essential Calm
- Mood Plus
- Exhilarin
- Adreset
- Brain Calm
- Brain Mood

- Relaxeze
- Relora Plex
- Sereniten Plus
- Satiet-Ease
- Blisphora
- Cortico B5B6

- Cortisol Manager
- Stress B Complex
- Licorice Plus
- MACA
- Rhodiola
- Trancor

The Thyroid Connection:
- Thyroid Support
- Thyroid PX
- Essential Thyroid
- Zinc citrate

- Vitamin A
- Vitamin D3/K2
- Selenomethionine-Selenium

Estrogen Dominance:
- DIM Enhanced
- Estro Apdapt
- Estromend
- Estrofactors
- Estro PX
- Progestomend

- Calcium D Glucarate
- LVDTX
- Liver Formula RX
- Fiber Formula
- Metafiber
- Medibulk

Food Allergies:
- L-glutamine
- Glutagenics
- BPP Enzymes
- Dipan-9
- Ultrazyme
- GI Digest

- Ultra Flora Balance
- HMF Intensive
- HMF Replenish
- HMF IBS
- HMF Replete
- Multi Encap

- Women's Nutrients
- Men's Nutrients
- Omega Plus
- Klean Omega

The Yeast Connection-Candida:
- Ultra Flora Balance
- HMF Intensive
- HMF Replenish
- HMF IBS
- HMF Replete
- HMF Antibiotic Care
- Sacro B
- Yeast Balance Complex
- Anti-MFP
- Caprylex
- Candida Terminator
- Paracide
- Candida Bactin-AR
- Berberine 500
- All above liver toxicity recommendations

Sleep:
- Benesom
- Nite Eze
- Essential Sleep/Ultra
- Pharm Gaba 250
- Griffonia
- Relaxeze
- Cortisol Manager
- Melatonin 3mg/5mg
- Melatonin PR (prolonged release)
- Brain Calm
- Theanine
- Brain Mood
- Essential Euphoria
- Trancor

Insulin Resistance:
- MetaglycemX
- Chromium picolinate
- Glucoplex
- ALA Max
- Antioxidant Synergy
- EPA 720/EPA 500
- Omega Plus
- Klean Omega

- Medibulk
- Metafiber
- Fiber Formula

Supplement Companies:

AOR

3900 – 12 Street NE

Calgary, AB T2E 8H9 Canada

www.aor.ca

Avicenna

North Vancouver, BC Canada

www.avicennanatural.com

Biotics

6801 Biotics Research Dr

Rosenberg, TX 77471

www.bioticsresearch.com

Boiron

1300 René-Descartes

Saint-Bruno-de-Montarville, QC J3V 0B7 Canada

www.boiron.ca

Douglas Labs

552 Newbold Street

London, ON N6E 2S5 Canada

www.douglaslabs.ca

Enzed Nutricorp

2402 Canoe Ave.

Coquitlam BC V3K 6C2

Canada

www.enzednaturals.com

Integrative Therapeutics

825 Challenger Drive

Green Bay, WI 54311 USA

www.integrativepro.com

Metagenics

100 Avenida La Pata

San Clemente, CA 92673 USA

www.metagenics.com

Oona

803 Washington St.

New York, NY 10014 USA

www.oonausa.com

Pascoe

Unit 70-40 Vogell Road

Richmond Hill, Ontario L4B 3N6 Canada

www.pascoecanada.com

Promedics

PO Box 155

2498 W 41st Avenue

Vancouver, BC V6M 2A7 Canada

www.promedics.ca

Restorative Formulations

93 Barre Street, Suite #1

Montpelier, VT 05602

www.restorativeformulations.com

Seroyal (Genestra)

490 Elgin Mills Road East

Richmond Hill, ON L4C 0L8 Canada

www.seroyal.com

Thorne Research, Inc.

P.O. Box 25

Dover, ID 83825 USA

www.thorne.com

Xymogen

6900 Kingspointe Pkwy.

Orlando, FL 32819

www.xymogen.com

100% Pure

2221 Oakland Road

San Jose, California 95131

www.100percentpure.ca

Appendix

Recommended Lab Testing

The following lab tests available through Dr Cobi:

- Comprehensive Female or Male Hormone Panel- ZRT Labs
- Sleep Balance Profile- ZRT Labs
- Complete Thyroid Panel-ZRT Labs
- Weight Management Panel- ZRT Labs
- CardioMetabolic Panel- ZRT Labs
- Adrenal Stress Index- Diagnostechs Labs
- GastroIntestinal Health Panel-Diagnostechs Labs
- ELISA Food Allergy Panel- Stero Chrom Laboratory

Recommended Labs:

ZRT Labs

8605 SW Creekside Place

Beaverton, OR 97008 USA

Diagnos-Techs

19110 66th S, Bldg G

Kent, WA 98032 USA

Stero Chrom Analytical

7825 Edmonds Street

Burnaby, BC V3N 1B9 Canada

Helpful Nutrition Websites

The following websites are a wealth of information and collectively contain thousands of healthy and delicious recipes:

- www.drcobi.com
- www.eatcleanmenus.com
- www.nourishingmeals.com
- www.wholelifenutrition.net
- www.againstallgrain.com
- www.thepaleomama.com
- www.paleogrubs.com
- www.detoxinista.com
- www.ohsheglows.com
- www.essentiallivingfoods.com
- www.simplysugarandglutenfree.com
- www.foodbabe.com

Bibliography

http://www.thealternativedaily.com/liver-toxicity-could-be-the-major-cause-of-your-weight-gain/

http://www.restorehealthcenter.net/blog/liver-weight-and-health/

http://www.wellnessresources.com/weight/articles/unclog_your_liver_lose_your_abdominal_fat_leptin_diet_weight_loss_challenge/

http://www.womentowomen.com/healthy-weight/weight-loss-and-adrenal-stress-2/

http://drhyman.com/blog/2010/04/20/are-your-food-allergies-making-you-fat/

http://www.foodallergyandglutenfreeweightloss.com/why_are_we_overweight.html

http://www.webmd.com/diet/sleep-and-weight-loss?page=2

http://www.huffingtonpost.com/susan-b-dopart-ms-rd/weight-loss-tips-are-your_b_598250.html

http://www.womentowomen.com/insulin-resistance/what-is-insulin-resistance/

http://weight.insulitelabs.com/Root-Cause-of-Insulin-Resistance.php

http://drhyman.com/blog/2010/05/20/5-steps-to-reversing-type-2-diabetes-and-insulin-resistance/

http://www.doctoroz.com/article/medications-may-cause-weight-gain?page=1

CPSIA information can be obtained
at www.ICGtesting.com
Printed in the USA
LVOW01s0816091215
465973LV00002B/6/P

9 781498 423243